Fertility and Obstetrics
in the Horse

LIBRARY OF VETERINARY PRACTICE

LIBRARY OF VETERINARY PRACTICE

Fertility and Obstetrics in the Horse

W. EDWARD ALLEN
MVB, PhD, FRCVS
Senior Lecturer in Animal Reproduction
Department of Surgery and Obstetrics
Royal Veterinary College
Hawkshead Lane
North Mymms
Hatfield, Herts

BLACKWELL SCIENTIFIC PUBLICATIONS

OXFORD LONDON EDINBURGH

BOSTON PALO ALTO MELBOURNE

©1988 by
Blackwell Scientific Publications
Editorial offices:
Osney Mead, Oxford OX2 OEL
    (*Orders*: Tel. 0865 240201)
8 John Street, London WCIN 2ES
23 Ainslie Place, Edinburgh EH3 6AJ
Three Cambridge Center, Suite 208,
    Cambridge, MA 02142, USA
667 Lytton Avenue, Palo Alto
    California 94301, USA
107 Barry Street, Carlton
    Victoria 3053, Australia

First published 1988

Set by Setrite Typesetters
Hong Kong
Printed and bound
in Great Britain by
Redwood Burn Limited,
Trowbridge, Wiltshire

DISTRIBUTORS

USA
    Year Book Medical Publishers
    200 North LaSalle Street
    Chicago, Illinois 60601
    (*Orders*: Tel. 312 726−9733)

Canada
    The C.V. Mosby Company
    5240 Finch Avenue East,
    Scarborough, Ontario
    (*Orders*: Tel. 416−298−1588)

Australia
    Blackwell Scientific Publications
    (Australia) Pty Ltd
    107 Barry Street
    Carlton, Victoria 3053
    (*Orders*: Tel. (03) 347 0300)

British Library
Cataloguing in Publication Data

Allen, W. Edward
    Fertility and obstetrics in the horse. —
    (Library of veterinary practice).
    1. Mares   2. Veterinary obstetrics
    I. Title   II. Series
    636.1'08982   SF959.U75

ISBN 0-632-02136-5

Contents

Preface   ix

1   Anatomy of the mare's genital system   1

1.1 Vulva; 1.2 Vestibule; 1.3 Vulvo-vaginal constriction; 1.4 Vagina;
1.5 Cervix uteri; 1.6 Uterus; 1.7 Broad ligaments; 1.8 Ovaries;
1.9 Uterine (Fallopian) tubes.

2   Endocrine control of the oestrous cycle and puberty   6

2.1 Definitions; 2.2 Hormonal changes; 2.3 Puberty

3   Clinical examination of the mare's genital system   9

3.1 Restraint of the mare; 3.2 Approach of the clinician; 3.3 External
examination; 3.4 Manual examination *per rectum*; 3.5 Ultrasound
examination *per rectum*; 3.6 Visual examination *per vaginam*; 3.7 Manual
examination *per vaginam*

4   Cyclical changes in the genital tract   18

4.1 Anoestrus; 4.2 Transition; 4.3 Oestrus; 4.4 Ovulation;
4.5 Development of corpus luteum; 4.6 Interoestrus; 4.7 Early
interoestrus versus early oestrus; 4.8 Prolonged dioestrus

5   Artificial control of cyclical activity   22

5.1 To shorten the transition between anoestrus and cyclic activity;
5.2 To shorten the luteal phase; 5.3 To hasten ovulation;
5.4 To synchronize ovulation

6   Teasing and covering procedure   25

6.1 Signs of oestrus; 6.2 Detection of oestrus; 6.3 Teasing technique;
6.4 Restraint of the mare for covering; 6.5 Injuries during covering

7   Normal pregnancy   30

7.1 Uterine changes; 7.2 Development of the conceptus; 7.3 Placenta
and fetal membranes; 7.4 Endocrine changes; 7.5 Cervical changes;
7.6 Ovarian changes; 7.7 Twinning; 7.8 Duration of pregnancy

8   Pregnancy diagnosis   39

8.1 Absence of subsequent oestrus; 8.2 Progesterone; 8.3 Clinical
examination; 8.4 Ultrasound scanning; 8.5 Equine chorionic
gonadotrophin; 8.6 Placental oestrogens

9 Normal parturition   44

9.1 Endocrine control; 9.2 Preparation of the environment; 9.3 The 'overdue' foal; 9.4 First stage labour; 9.5 Second stage labour; 9.6 Third stage labour; 9.7 Induction of parturition

10 Post-partum events   50

10.1 Uterine involution; 10.2 Post-partum infection; 10.3 The foal heat

11 Normal expectations of fertility   52

11.1 Conception and foaling rates; 11.2 Effect of management on fertility; 11.3 Methods of investigating reproductive function in mares

12 Non-infectious infertility in mares   55

12.1 Prolonged dioestrus; 12.2 Erratic behaviour early in the season; 12.3 Erratic post-partum behaviour; 12.4 Silent heat; 12.5 Split oestrus; 12.6 Failure of corpus luteum formation; 12.7 Cystic ovaries *do not* occur in the mare; 12.8 Nymphomania; 12.9 Granulosa cell tumour; 12.10 Chromosome abnormalities; 12.11 Abnormalities of the uterine tubes; 12.12 Uterine cysts; 12.13 Partial dilation of the uterus; 12.14 Lesions of the cervix; 12.15 Persistent hymen; 12.16 Vaginal bleeding

13 Infectious infertility   63

13.1 General considerations; 13.2 Non specific infections; 13.3 Pyometra; 13.4 Venereal bacteria

14 Swabbing techniques and diagnosis of endometritis   71

14.1 Clitoral swabbing; 14.2 Uterine swabbing; 14.3 Processing the swab; 14.4 Endometrial biopsy

15 Treatment and prevention of endometritis   82

15.1 General consideration; 15.2 Mares with impaired uterine resistance; 15.3 Chronic endometritis; 15.4 Uro-vagina; 15.5 Cystic endometritis; 15.6 Pyometra; 15.7 Post-partum metritis; 15.8 Pneumovagina; 15.9 Local clitoral treatment; 15.10 Clitoral sinusectomy

16 Viral causes of infertility   88

16.1 Viral abortion; 16.2 Coital exanthema; 16.3 Viral arteritis

17 Problems during pregnancy   89

17.1 Definitions in pregnancy development; 17.2 Resorption; 17.3 Mummification; 17.4 Abortion; 17.5 Pseudopregnancy; 17.6 Pregnancy failure

18   Causes of pregnancy failure   94
     18.1 Bacterial infection; 18.2 Viral infection; 18.3 Twinning;
     18.4 Miscellaneous

19   Other abnormal events during pregnancy   99
     19.1 Uterine torsion; 19.2 Ventral hernia; 19.3 Pseudopregnancy

20   Reducing infertility caused by twin pregnancy   101
     20.1 Prevention of twin conception; 20.2 Diagnosis of twins;
     20.3 Dealing with twin conception

21   Retained placenta   104
     21.1 Normal expulsion; 21.2 Examination of the membranes;
     21.3 Abnormal expulsion

22   Other post-partum problems   110
     22.1 Vulval and perineal trauma; 22.2 Recto-vaginal fistula;
     22.3 Perineal laceration; 22.4 Ruptures of the cervix and vagina *per se*;
     22.5 Uterine rupture; 22.6 Haematoma; 22.7 Uterine prolapse;
     22.8 Hypocalcaemia; 22.9 Post-partum endometritis;
     22.10 Management of the engorged udder

23   Manipulation of reproduction   114
     23.1 Artificial insemination; 23.2 Embryo transfer; 23.3 Manipulation
     of embryos

24   Dystocia   118
     24.1 Definitions; 24.2 Significance of dystocia; 24.3 Recognition of
     dystocia; 24.4 Non-surgical treatment of dystocia; 24.5 Surgical
     treatment of dystocia

25   The normal stallion   125
     25.1 Anatomy; 25.2 Endocrine control; 25.3 Physiology of sperm
     production; 25.4 Covering behaviour

26   Examination of the stallion for breeding soundness   136
     26.1 Bacteriological swabbing; 26.2 Physical examination; 26.3 Semen
     collection; 26.4 Semen evaluation

27   Infertility in the stallion   144
     27.1 Poor semen quality; 27.2 Infections; 27.3 Physical abnormalities;
     27.4 Psychological problems

28   Miscellaneous   151
     28.1 Breeding terms; 28.2 The 'riggy' gelding; 28.3 Stallion 'vices';
     28.4 'Hidden' costs at stud; 28.5 Rectal tears

     Appendix   159

     Further reading   168

     Index   169

Preface

This book was written mainly with a view to describing the diagnostic procedures and treatment techniques commonly used in the routine management of brood mares and the reasons for their application; attention is drawn to those areas where knowledge is scant, and where popular belief appears to be misinformed.

Whilst recommending what is considered to be ideal, the author has also tried to comment on what may be practical, given that the cost of veterinary help can be prohibitive for some mare owners and inconsequential for others (stud fees vary from less than £50 to over £100,000). Any book of this nature must in general reflect the views of the author, although attention has been drawn to alternative opinions as often as possible. In particular, however, the author is extremely grateful for the advice of a long-time and good friend, John R. Newcombe, BVetMed, MRCVS, who probably examines more brood mares each year than any other veterinary surgeon in the United Kingdom.

The assistance of Barbara Robertson was also invaluable; she typed the manuscript from mainly unintelligible writing which was penned with a gift from the author's children, Aisling and Ralph. John Sutton, JP, MRCVS, has been an extremely patient and understanding editor, and David Gunn prepared the illustrations. Appendix 1 is reproduced by permission of the editor of the *Veterinary Record*.

The author has written this book primarily with veterinary undergraduates in mind, but hopes that it will contain information of interest to veterinary surgeons in practice. Additionally both mare and stallion owners may find the answers to some of the vexing problems which they encounter when breeding their horses; they may also appreciate the complexity of the reproductive process in the horse and be more tolerant with mares that fail to produce a foal and with the people who have participated in this lack of success.

W.E.A.

1 / Anatomy of the mare's genital system

1.1 Vulva

- lies below the anus (at risk from contamination by faeces)
- normally almost vertical with firmly closed lips (**15.5**).

1.2 Vestibule

- extends from vulval lips to vestibulo-vaginal constriction
- ventrally houses the clitoris which is surrounded laterally and ventrally by clitoral fossa
- the dorsal surface of the clitoris contains up to three small cavities, the clitoral sinuses (**14.1**).

1.3 Vulvo-vaginal constriction

- just anterior to urethral opening
- may be partial remnants or complete hymen at this junction in maiden mares
- in genitally healthy mares this constriction forms a secondary line of defence against aspirated air and faecal material.

1.4 Vagina

- a potentially hollow tube which when undisturbed is completely collapsed
- not palpable *per rectum*
- most of the vagina is retroperitoneal.

1.5 Cervix uteri

- a tubular organ 1–7 cm long
- last line of defence between uterine lumen and atmosphere
- the length, diameter, tone and patency of the cervix varies greatly during different reproductive states (**4.1**–**4.8**)
- at no time in the normal mare is the cervix so tightly closed that it cannot be dilated manually

• part of the cervix projects caudally into the potential cavity of the vagina, and its appearance is useful for determining the mare's reproductive status.

1.6   Uterus

• roughly T or Y shaped and consists of a body and two horns (Fig. 1.1)
• the body runs forward and downwards on the anterior floor of the pelvis, and caudal abdomen, dorsal or dorso-lateral to the bladder
• the horns bifurcate from the cranial end of the body, and run laterally, or dorso-laterally
• the normal non-pregnant uterus has a potential lumen
• the thickness of the uterine walls, and the tone of the myometrium, vary with the reproductive state and age
• pregnancy causes gross distortion of the shape of the uterus (**7.1**).

1.7   Broad ligaments

• each one extends from the dorso-caudal border of a horn, and the dorso-lateral border of the body to the sublumbar and lateral pelvic wall
• distal to the uterine horns they suspend, and expand to cover, the ovaries.

1.8   Ovaries

• bean shaped, but shape and size quite variable dependent mainly on follicular content (**4.1−4.8, 7.6**) (Fig. 1.2)
• resting (anoestrus) size ranges from $4 \times 2 \times 2$ cm to $8 \times 4 \times 4$ cm, tend to be largest in older and larger mares
• suspended in the antero-lateral part of the broad ligament (the mesovarium)
• the broad ligament between the ovary and tip of uterine horn is the utero-ovarian ligament
• the ovary is covered by an extension of the broad ligament (serosa) except at the ovulation fossa, which is a marked depression on its antero-medial border

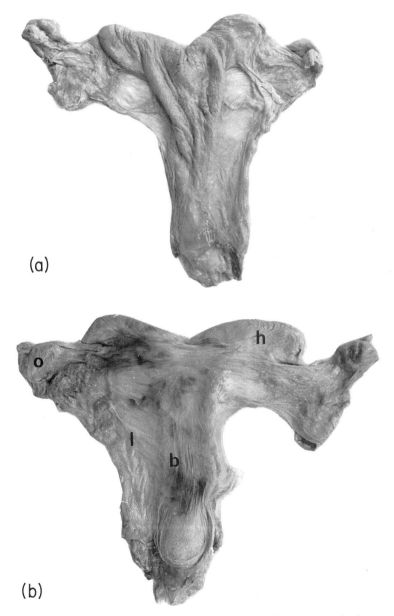

Fig. 1.1. (a) Ventral surface of uterus. (b) Dorsal surface of uterus: **h**, uterine horn; **b**, uterine body; **o**, ovary; **l**, broad ligament.

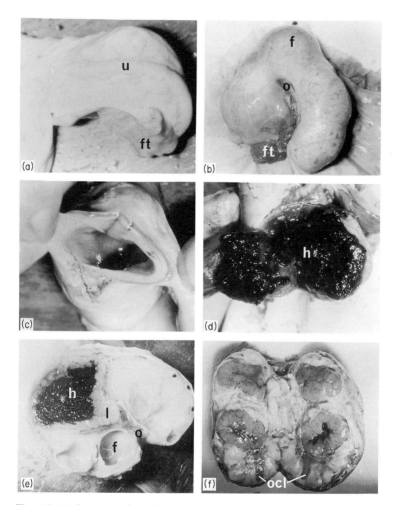

Fig. 1.2. (a) Lateral surface of ovary covered by mesosalpynx containing uterine tube. (b) Medial surface of ovary showing ovulation fossa. (c) Mature follicle opened to show fluid filled cavity. (d) Corpus haemorrhagicum sectioned to show extensive haematoma. (e)Formalin preserved ovary sectioned to show developing corpus luteum with central haematoma. (f) Sectioned ovary containing two mature corpora lutea, one of which has a central haematoma; the corpus luteum of the previous cycle has not yet turned yellow. **u**, uterine tube; **o**, ovulation fossa; **f**, follicle; **ft**, fibriae of uterine tube; **h**, haematoma; **l**, luteal tissue; **ocl**, old corpus luteum.

• large variations in size, shape and consistency occur in normal mares.

1.9   Uterine (Fallopian) tubes

• run from tip of uterine horn to ovary in a fold of the broad ligament (the mesosalpinx)
• uterine end (isthmus) opens at the tip of the horn on a small papilla
• ovarian end (ampulla) terminates in distinct fimbriae which are partially attached to the serosal covering of the ovary adjacent to the ovulation fossa.

2 / Endocrine control of the oestrous cycle and puberty

2.1 Definitions

Cycle length

This is the interval between two successive oestrous ovulations (but may get double ovulations during same heat or dioestrous ovulations); this is a more accurate mesurement than beginning of one heat to beginning of next. Cycle length usually ±21 days but is very variable. Longest in spring. If shorter than 19 days suspect endometritis (**13.1**). Abnormal persistence if corpus luteum (**CL**) = prolonged dioestrus, i.e. long cycle (**4.8**).

Anoestrus

Prolonged period of ovarian inactivity. May be small follicles in ovaries. No functional CL. Usually winter and spring, depending on mare and management. Occasionally in summer, especially in lactating mare and in type II pseudopregnancy (**17.5**), cf. prolonged dioestrus and pregnancy.

Transitions from anoestrus to regular cycles

Winter or spring, depending on mare and management. Variable follicular activity with many follicles becoming atretic; erratic oestrous behaviour. Oestrus may last more than a month before the first ovulation occurs.

Oestrus

Period of acceptance of stallion. Usually 4−7 days but very variable. Longest in spring (i.e. first heat of year); usually ends ±24 hours after ovulation. Under endocrine and psychological control. But split-oestrus, silent heat, shy breeders, nymphomania (**12.4**, **12.5**, **12.8**).

Interoestrus

Roughly synonymous with dioestrus, but more accurately describes the interval between two successive heats. Usually 14−16 days, but longest after early heats in year. May be short if CL lysed due to endometritis (**13.1**) or after prostaglandin (PG) administration (**5.2**). Prolonged due to persistence of CL (prolonged dioestrus) (**4.8**).

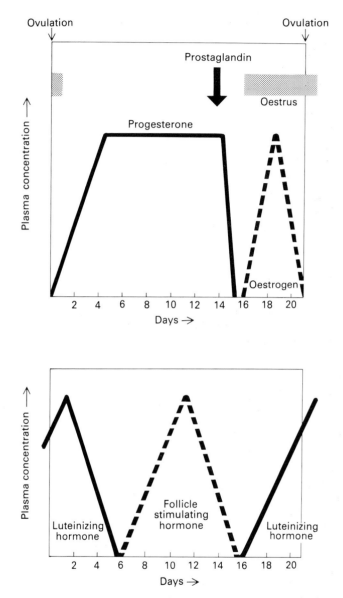

Fig. 2.1. Diagramatic representation of the major hormonal events in the mare's oestrous cycle.

Luteal phase
Ovulation to luteolysis, i.e. 14 or 15 days. Shortened by endometritis or PG administration (after day 5). Short luteal phase may shorten interoestrus but not always, especially in spring. Corpus luteum may not lyse spontaneously for up to 3 months (prolonged dioestrus).

2.2 Hormonal changes

The cycle is controlled by five major hormones (Fig. 2.1).
• Follicle stimulating hormone (FSH) from anterior pituitary gland. Peak blood concentrations in mid-dioestrus stimulate initial follicular growth (not usually palpable in ovaries). Low concentrations during oestrus
• Luteinizing hormone (LH) from anterior pituitary gland. Circulating levels low in late luteal phase. Start to rise in early oestrus and reach peak levels after ovulation. In the mare this hormone stimulates major follicular growth, maturation and ovulation. Values decrease as progesterone concentrations (from developing CL) rise
• Progesterone. Secreted by corpus haemorrhagicum (**4.5**) and corpus luteum. Blood concentrations start to rise after ovulation and reach a peak 5 days later. During this time the developing CL is refractory to prostaglandin (**5.2**). High levels of progesterone maintained until day 14 or 15, when CL is usually lysed by endogenous PG. CL persists spontaneously in prolonged dioestrus and pregnancy.
• Prostaglandin $F_2\alpha$ released from endometrium 13 to 15 days after ovulation. Enters general circulation and if quantities reaching CL are sufficient, causes luteolysis. Endometritis and intrauterine manipulation during luteal phase cause premature PG release (**13.1**)
• Oestrogens. Oestradiol $17-\beta$ and conjugated oestrogens, especially oestrone sulphate. Concentrations low during most of cycle but rise in early oestrus to reach peak values 48 hours before ovulation.

2.3 Puberty

Usually reached by 2 years, but some mares are ovulating as yearlings, especially if born early in the year. Puberty delayed by being in training and administration of anabolic steroids. Occasionally not achieved until 4 years in thoroughbreds. Turner's syndrome (**12.10**) may be mistaken for immaturity.

3 / Clinical examination of the mares' genital system

Basic examination of the genital tract consists of:
- visual examination of the perineum, vulva and tail
- manual palpation of the cervix, uterus and ovaries *per rectum*
- visual inspection of the vagina and cervix *per vaginam* using a speculum
- manual palpation of the vagina and cervix *per vaginam*
- the use of real time ultrasound, *per rectum*, is becoming more popular and makes examination more accurate (for other methods of examination see **11.3**)

3.1   Restraint of the mare

- Amount of restraint needed depends on experience, and temperament of mare, and quality and quantity of help available. Examination is most difficult in young undisciplined mares handled by amateurs, and easiest in old brood mares handled by experienced personnel. The presence of a foal at foot makes examination of most mares more difficult. No method of restraint is ideal.
- Temperament of mare. Some mares are vicious and kick when handled behind; these are uncommon. Most mares are apprehensive when examined the first time and may need more restraint than subsequently. Most mares tend to walk forward or move sideways if only loosely restrained during examination. The presence (or absence) of the mare's foal, or separation from a companion may make the mare uneasy, as can the sight of unfamiliar objects (clinician's protective clothing, coloured sleeves, lubricant bottles etc.). Examining mares in a field is made more difficult and more dangerous by the presence of other inquisitive horses.

Stocks
Probably the best method of restraint but:
- mare may not enter easily, especially for first time
- mare may be uneasy about being confined, especially initially
- mare may try to jump out, especially to join a companion or foal (it may be possible to put the foal in the stocks with the mare)

- ensure that the back panel of the stocks is low
- stocks should be readily dismantleable as occasionaly mares become cast.

Twitch

Very useful method of restraint and may be only form necessary for most mares, but:

- some owners resent application of twitch to their mare
- some mares are very difficult to twitch
- some mares won't move when twitched, so position correctly beforehand
- some mares try to go down when twitched tightly
- twitch will not always control a wilful mare
- humane twitch (Fig. 3.1) is easy to apply and leaves no mark on the nose. Not suitable for ponies (nose is too small).

Bridle

May be used with twitch or other methods. Helps the handler to stop the mare moving forward; a chiffney bit gives best control.

Bales

Bales of hay or straw behind the mare give some degree of protection against kicks, but:

- mare may resent presence of bales
- mare may take a step forward during initial examination.

Other methods of restraint

Lifting a front leg, on the side of the examiner stops the mare from kicking with the ipsilateral back leg, but:

- the clinician may have to stand directly behind the mare
- the back end of the mare tends to be lowered, which makes rectal examination particularly difficult
- an inexperienced helper may suddenly release the forelimb, or take too much of the mare's weight so that she can still kick.

Turning the mare's head towards the examiner helps to prevent her kicking with the hind leg on that same side.

Hind-leg hobbles help to prevent kicking but are seldom used in the UK.

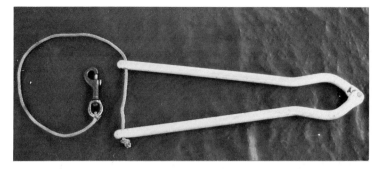

Fig. 3.1. Humane twitch.

Tranquilizers are not usually advisable because they may make the mare too unsteady.

3.2   Approach of clinician

Avoid sudden movements and loud noises, but try to converse with helper in an even voice, or hum or whistle.

When mare is not in stocks, approach her from the side, put one hand on the back, run it to base of the tail, grasp tail and pull it to one side.

• at this stage, mare's temperament and effectiveness of restraint will become apparent

• feel for discharge (wet or dried) on tail, and inspect perineum (**13.1, 15.5**)

• For manual examination *per rectum* or *vaginam*, the arm can be inserted initially without the operator standing directly behind the mare. As examination proceeds, more of the clinician's body is behind the mare, but at this stage her likely reaction has been anticipated

• for speculum examination *per vaginam*, it is most convenient for an assistant to hold the tail (in a gloved hand) to allow the clinician a free hand to part the vulval lips.

Round the door-post approach, with the mare against the wall. This is not advisable as:

• mare may resent initial positioning

• if mare steps forward during initial examination, clinician becomes exposed.

Examination over half-door not recommended except for clitoral swabbing (**14.1**).

Standing mare in a door-way with the back half in the yard is ideal for quiet mares (with or without twitch) which are accustomed to being examined. A light outside the box aids in speculum examination and protection to ultrasound equipment but a screen is more difficult to visualize. It may be difficult to persuade the mare to stop halfway through the doorway.

3.3 External examination

This may reveal:
• normal vulva — nearly perpendicular, no distortions (scarring) or discharges.
• sunken anus (due to old age, poor condition) common in thoroughbreds and causes antero-dorsal displacement of dorsal commisure of the vulva. This encourages contamination of the vulva and vestibule with faeces and predisposes to pneumovagina (**13.2**).
• vulva already sutured (Caslick's operation) to prevent pneumovagina.
• lateral or dorsal tears to vulva.
• small vesicles or ulcerated areas due to coital exanthema (herpes virus 3 — **16.2**). Not to be confused with small depigmented areas which are common.
• vulval discharge. Varies from sticky moistness at ventral commisure to frank discharge (wet or dried) on thighs and tail (**13.1**). A small amount of moisture is normal during oestrus, especially after covering.
• yellow urine stain (usually dry) on ventral commisure of vulva. Usually denotes oestrus (but not always present) — due to increased urinary frequency when showing (winking) (**4.3**).

3.4 Manual examination *per rectum*

• due to the lateral position of the ovaries, one-handed rectal examination makes accurate palpation of the right ovary for the right-handed examiner (and vice versa) difficult if the mare is not well restrained.
• wear a glove and use adequate lubricant.
• mare usually resents passage of hand most and then maybe elbow.

- evacuate rectum of faeces totally and feel for uterine horns lying transversely in front of pubis. Follow these laterally to ovaries which are in front of shaft of ileum.
- always try to have hand anterior to structure to be palpated to allow sufficient rectum for manipulation.
- do not stretch rectum laterally if tense or resist strong peristaltic contractions — otherwise rectum may tear (especially dorsally, i.e. not adjacent to examiner's hand) (**28.5**).
- if rectum is ballooned with air, feel forward for peristaltic constriction and gently stroke with finger to stimulate contraction.
- ovaries often lie lateral to broad ligament and are difficult to palpate. They must be manipulated onto antero-medial aspect of ligament for accurate palpation.
- uterus is very difficult to palpate in anoestrus, easier during cycles, and easiest during early (up to 60 days) pregnancy, due to increasing thickness and tension (tone) of the uterine wall (**4.1, 4.3, 7.1**).
- cervix is palpated by sweeeping finger tips ventrally from side to side in mid pelvic area. It is easiest to feel in luteal phases, but more difficult during oestrus and anoestrus (**4.1, 4.3, 4.6**).

3.5   Ultrasound examination *per rectum*

- real time linear array ultrasound allows the visualization of the ovaries and uterus and their contents; in particular fluid is easy to recognize
- machines in current use consist of a hand held probe (transducer) which is inserted into the mare's rectum; the transducer is connected to a visual display unit by a cable.
- the image on the VDU can be frozen, areas of interest can be measured and the picture can be photographed.
- very simply the moving picture is produced by the transducer emitting series of rapid pulses of high frequency ultrasound (3−7 mHz); for examination of the mare's genital tract a 5.0 mHz probe gives adequate penetration and optimal resolution.
- the sound waves are reflected by dense tissue, e.g. bone and the echo is received by the transducer and displayed as white on the screen.
- ultrasound passes through liquid without any reflections; this looks black on the screen and allows the identification of follicular fluid, fetal fluids, cysts and exudate (Figs 3.2 and 3.3).

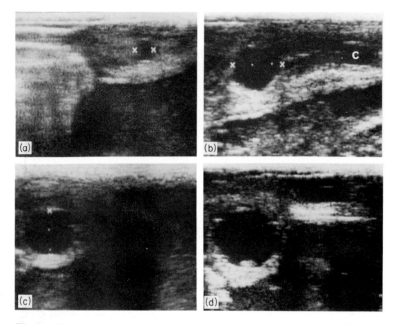

Fig. 3.2. Real-time ultrasonographic changes during early pregnancy (3 MHz linear array transducer). (a) 14 day pregnancy (x.x) in anterior uterine body. (b) 16 day pregnancy (x.x) in anterior uterine body; note cyst, **c**, in posterior body. (c) 16 day pregnancy (x.x) in uterine horn. (d) 22 day pregnancy; note embryo apparently attached to ventral wall. (e) 34 day pregnancy with dorsally situated embryo (x.x). (f) 37 day pregnancy with descending fetus (x.x). (g) 48 day pregnancy with fetus (x.x) on ventral wall of uterus; note parts of the umbilical cord dorsal to the fetus. (h) 53 day pregnancy. The head of the fetus is on the right, and limbs can be seen.

- most tissues reflect some ultrasound and therefore most of the screen looks grey; with experience different structures in the uterus and ovaries can be identified.
- the mare is restrained as for manual examination, with due regard to the safety of the machine.
- the screen is best viewed in subdued lighting, but this may be difficult to achieve.

3.6   Visual examination *per vaginam*

- requires optimal restraint, as operator will have to stand behind mare

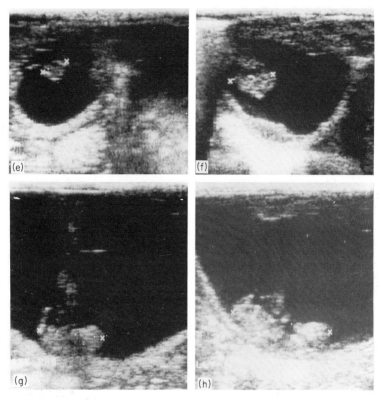

Fig. 3.2. (*contd*).

- clean perineum and vulva with clean water or disinfectant
- moisten or lubricate speculum
- after introducing speculum through vulval lips, push antero-dorsally to clear brim of pubis
- at this point there is often considerable resistance at vestibulo-vaginal junction (occasionally the speculum tries to enter the urethra)
- when fully inserted (±30 cm) view vaginal walls and cervix.

Types of speculum (see also uterine swabbing, **14.2**)

1 *Metal*, e.g. Russian duck-billed. Good visualization but cumbersome and difficult to clean. It requires a separate light source which must be protected.

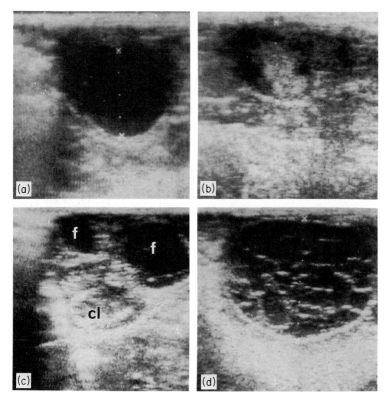

Fig. 3.3. Real-time ultrasonographic changes in the ovary and uterus (3 MHz linear array transducer). (a) Ovarian follicle (x.x). (b) Early (solid grey) corpus haemorhagicum surrounded by small (black) follicles. (c) Older corpus luteum, **cl** and two follicles, **f**. (d) Luteinized follicle which did not ovulate. (e) Uterine oedema in endometrial folds during oestrus. There is a small amount of fluid, **e**, in the lumen (5 mHz transducer). (f) Uterine fluid during dioestrus (3.5 mHz transducer). (g) Copious uterine exudate (x.x), i.e. pyometra; the fluid may be clear as in this case or turbid. (h) Twin pregnancies, one at the base of each horn. The fetus on the right died spontaneously at about day 38.

2   *Plastic*. Replaceable tubular speculum with integral light source. If vagina does not balloon with air, cervix is difficult to visualize. Reduces likelihood of spreading venereal infection. Difficult to visualize dorsal wall of vagina (recto-vaginal fistula, **13.2**). Light source often temperamental.

3   *Cardboard*. tubular with silvered interior to reflect light. Requires

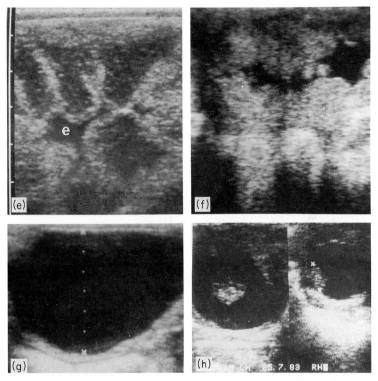

Fig. 3.3. (*contd*).

separate light source. Slightly longer than plastic speculum but disposable and cheap — avoids resterilization.

3.7 Manual examination *per vaginam*

- clean vulva and insert lubricated gloved hand
- may feel remnants of hymen — occasionally complete (**12.15**)
- vagina dry in luteal phase and anoestrus, moist in oestrus
- palpate cervix for shape, size and patency of canal
- may detect adhesions or fibrosis (**12.14**)
- do not force finger along cervical canal if there is a possibility of pregnancy
- mares cervix will allow gentle dilation without causing damage, at all stages of reproduction
- manual examination may not be possible if mare's vulva is stitched excessively tight (**13.2**)

4 / Cyclical changes in genital tract

4.1 Anoestrus

- ovaries: small, hard, bean shaped, may be small follicles
- uterus: thin walled and flaccid, may be difficult to palpate
- vagina: pale and dry
- cervix:
 (i) dry, pale and looks closed (speculum).
 (ii) dry, short and easily admits two fingers but may be tighter in maiden and older mares (palpation *per vaginam*)
 (iii) soft, wide and difficult to palpate per rectum.

4.2 Transition

- ovaries: become softer, follicles grow (3–5 cm) then regress. May be repeated waves of follicles. Difficult to anticipate which follicle will ovulate and when. Ovulation usually followed by regular, ovulatory cycles
- uterus: flaccid or slight tone
- vagina: depends on ovarian contents, i.e. from typically anoestrus to typically oestrus.
- cervix: cervix remains soft and difficult to palpate *per rectum*; changes noted *per vaginam* depend on ovarian contents.

4.3 Oestrus

- ovaries: usually follicles 2–3 cm on first day. One or more grow to 4–6 cm before ovulation; sometimes smaller follicles will ovulate, especially in small ovaries. Follicles are black (non-echogenic) on ultrasound examination. Oestrus ends 0–2 days after ovulation
- uterus: endometrial folds enlarge and become oedematous — uterus feels thickened, heavier and 'doughy' but not tonic; oedema and uterine folds can be seen on ultrasound — these are most marked two days before ovulation
- vagina: progressively more moist and hyperaemic
- cervix:
 (i) moist, hyperaemic, folds oedematous and cervix appears to rest on floor of vagina (speculum).

(ii) moist, $\pm$ 4 cm long, admits 1–2 fingers (more at foal heat) feels oedematous; may contract when palpated *per vaginam*.

(iii) *per rectum* feels soft when fully relaxed. In some mares soft anteriorly and hard posteriorly, but shorter than dioestrus.

• vulva: may relax more during oestrus in some mares — not consistent. Sometimes a yellow stain on ventral commisure due to frequent urination.

NB, cervical relaxation may be poor in maiden and older mares.

4.4   Ovulation

Accurate detection important as:
• confirms that ovulation has occurred
• confirms time of ovulation relative to service
• may identify multiple ovulations; this is easy using ultrasound examination (**18.3, 20.1–20.3**).

Accurate detection can only be achieved by daily palpation of ovaries. Ovulation always occurs at ovulation fossa (Fig. 1.2). Mature follicles are softer, and just before ovulation may become very soft and tender; distortion of the shape of the follicle can be seen at this time with ultrasound examination.

• occasionally follicles collapse during palpation of the ovary — this does not affect fertility; it is difficult and inadvisable to try to burst follicles manually.

• during ovulation follicular fluid and ovum are released (fimbriae of the fallopian tube cover the fossa at this time to collect ovum). After ovulation the follicle is collapsed. The part of the ovary that contained it feels very soft and the ovary is usually tender when palpated (mare twitches flank, looks at flank or kicks at belly). Some mares resent being saddled.

• after about 12 hours haemorrhage redistends follicle cavity, i.e. it forms corpus haemorrhagicum (CH); this is usually about 3/4s of the size of the original follicle but may be similar sized or occasionally very large (10–15 cm — this structure functions as normal CH and CL but may remain palpable for weeks).

• CH (and developing CL) may be impossible to distinguish from a follicle on one examination. If palpable structure is not spherical, i.e. flattened in one dimension or discus-like it is not a follicle. Ultrasound shows up formed elements (thrombus) in CH, which are intensely white.

4.5   Development of corpus luteum (from CH)

This takes 4−6 days, but progesterone production starts immediately. The maturing corpus luteum becomes *smaller* and firmer due to:
• shrinkage of the thrombus, which is also being invaded by:
• rapidly dividing peripheral (thecal) cells which become luteal cells (produce progesterone), and
• condensation of ovarian stroma which becomes thicker round CL due to its diminished surface area. This results in CL usually not being palpable in the ovary 4−5 days after ovulation. CLs which form from large CHs remain palpable and visible longest.

4.6   Interoestrus (dioestrus)

• ovaries: CH may be palpable for some days and detectable by ultrasound until after regression has started; one ovary is bigger than the other. Occasionally follicles are present during the luteal phase, more often prior to oestrus. Rarely ovulations (dioestrous) occur during the luteal phase
• uterus: becomes more tonic (tubular) especially in the late luteal phase. Uterine changes are not palpably consistent and vary greatly between mares
• cervix:
  (i) dry, pale and projects into a distended vaginal lumen (speculum).
  (ii) dry, finger-like and difficult to locate external os on palpation. (NB, normal mare's cervix will always dilate to accommodate a finger, even during pregnancy.)
  (iii) Firm and tubular *per rectum*, i.e. ±8 cm long and one centimetre wide.

4.7   Early interoestrus versus early oestrus (early heat)

It is often impossible to distinguish between these two phases at one examination as:
• small follicles are difficult to distinguish from early CL without ultrasound
• uterine condition is not diagnostic
• the cervix takes 2−4 days to change from luteal to oestrous and vice versa.

4.8 Prolonged dioestrus (persistent CL)

- ovaries: CL not palpable. Usually follicles are present, increasing in number and size with increased length of dioestrus. Some of these follicles ovulate
- uterus: usually becomes more tubular and tense (tonic) with increased length of dioestrus (cf, early pregnancy)
- cervix: similar to late luteal phase and early pregnancy.

5 / Artificial control of cyclical activity

5.1   To shorten the transition between anoestrous and cyclic activity

• i.e. to produce an ovulatory oestrus by mid February — this usually involves providing artificial light and treatment with a hormone (allyltrenbolone) in the food for 10–16 days
• plan ahead
• provide light for a minimum of 16 hours daily, e.g. 7 am–11 pm — alternatively leave lights on all night
• good quality light, i.e. 150 watt *clear* bulb in centre of 12' × 12' box or 4' (40 watt) strip light is essential.
• ideally there should be light falling upon the eyes wherever the horse stands — avoid shadows cast by beams or partitions; high dark ceilings reflect very little light
• it should be easy to read a newspaper wherever you stand in the box
• if the light intensity is insufficient there is no response
• mares commencing the lighting regime in poor bodily condition take longer to respond than those in good condition; the aim is to increase the level of nutrition and consequently the mare's condition
• it is just as important to ensure that mares already in good or fat condition are sufficiently well fed to maintain their body weight
• the length of time taken from beginning the regime to ovulation (response time) is affected by several factors:

(i) Initial condition of mare and rate of improvement.

(ii) Time of year; regime started early March probably 'works' about 2 weeks faster than if started in December/January.

(iii) Individual mare variation; occasionally mares are very slow to respond whilst others begin spontaneous ovulation several weeks earlier than would be expected.

The 'response time' can be shortened by the use of allyltrenbolone (a progestagen). The stage at which the course of treatment is started is relatively critical:

(i) If started in deep anoestrus with no pre-lighting, the mare will remain anoestrus.

(ii) If started in shallow anoestrus with insufficient pre-lighting, the mare will come into season with follicular growth but without ovulation and will then return to anoestrus.

(iii) If started in shallow anoestrus, after 4–6 weeks of 'lights' or in prolonged oestrus in late March or early April then ovulation should result.

(iv) If started in prolonged oestrus from January to March without prelighting then ovulation will probably not occur.

(v) If started in prolonged oestrus mid-April or later then the first ovulation could have occurred earlier without treatment.

• it appears that those mares which fail to ovulate after allyltrenbolone treatment return to a deeper anoestrus than might be expected, so that eventual ovulation, whether spontaneous or following another course, is later than would have otherwise occurred

• ovulation occurs 'classically' around 10 days after the last dose of allyltrenbolone but this interval is very variable. Some mares enter prolonged oestrus, eventually ovulating after 3 or 4 weeks

• treament starting in January and February often results in ovulation about 15 days after the last dose

• courses given in April may result in ovulation within 7 days, but if a large follicle was present at the beginning of the course it may:

(i) ovulate during the course.

(ii) ovulate within 24–48 hours of the end of the course (with or without oestrus).

(iii) regress.

• occasionally a small follicle may grow during allyltrenbolone treatment and then ovulate within 24–48 hours of the end

• for all these reasons it is advisable to examine the mare on or about the last day of treatment

• during the course of allyltrenbolone treatment FSH stimulates the initial growth and 'priming' of small follicles; LH concentrations in plasma are low

• after termination of successful treatment, LH concentrations rise and cause follicular maturation and ovulation.

5.2   To shorten the luteal phase

• i.e. of normal dioestrus, prolonged dioestrus and pregnancy up to 35 days (**17.2, 20.3**)

• prostaglandin (one dose is usually sufficient) causes prompt luteolysis and subsequent ovulation in 4–10 days, but:

• prolonged dioestrus — if large follicles are present (**4.8**) one may ovulate rapidly (24−48 hours after treatment) without the mare showing signs of heat, or she may be in oestrus for only 12−36 hours after ovulation
• young corpus luteum (< 6 days) will not respond to prostaglandin
• if the mare has had dioestrus ovulation (i.e. now has two CLs) the youngest CL may not respond
• may cause sweating, transient diarrhoea and occasionally colicy signs
• mares with chronic obstructive pulmonary disease may exhibit respiratory embarrassment
• occasionally exogenous PG will not cause luteolysis; it is then necessary to dilate the cervix and irrigate the uterus with 250−500 ml warm saline. This may cause transient discharge.

5.3   To hasten ovulation

• hCG (human chorionic gonadotrophin — 'holding injection') is given when a follicle of 4 cm or larger is present. Ovulation usually occurs within 48 hours, but:
• rarely do mares have an anaphylactic reaction to hCG
• no guarantee that the mare will conceive. hCG only hastens ovulation, thus avoiding repeated coverings
• gonadotrophin releasing hormone (GnRH) is of limited value in inducing ovulation in mares.
NB. The efficacy of any treatment designed to stimulate ovulation is difficult to assess as the drug is given at a time when ovulation would be expected anyway.

5.4   Synchronizing ovulation

• e.g. for embryo transfer or batch artificial insemination
• many different methods are available, e.g:
• oral allyltrenbolone for 14 days, prostaglandin on day 7 to lyse any luteal tissue; hCG 4 or 5 days after allyltrenbolone withdrawal.

6 / Teasing and covering procedure

6.1 Signs of oestrus

Mares vary in their willingness to show oestrus both from day to day, heat to heat and mare to mare. This may be influenced by teasing procedure.

• some mares show readily to other mares and people, some show only to male horses and some will not show at all (**12.4, 12.5**).
Classical signs are:

• the mare straddles hind legs, raises tail, crouches slightly, urinates and persistently everts her clitoris (winking or showing)
• some mares may 'wink' without urinating or lifting tail
• other mares are just less aggressive when teased
• mares rarely mount each other but occasionally mares in advanced pregnancy will mount mares in heat
• many shy or bad tempered mares show better when twitched
• maiden mares often 'show' well but are difficult to cover without restraint
• some mares with foals show best when the foal is present, others when it is out of earshot
• mares not in heat are either indifferent (especially in anoestrus) or violent, i.e. kick, bite, buck or strike out.

6.2 Detection of oestrus

This may be by:
• seeing mare show spontaneously to an object, the owner or another horse
• change of temperament — but this is often misleading, i.e. owner thinks the mare is in heat when she is not
• slight stickyness or yellow stain at ventral commisure of vulva
• some people can smell a mare in heat
• clinical examination by veterinary surgeon
• using a teaser, e.g.:
 (i) the stallion by which the mare is to be covered
 (ii) teaser stallion kept for the purpose — cheaper to keep and easier to manage, especially if a pony is used
 (iii) gelding that is 'riggy'

(iv) gelding that has been hormone (testosterone or oestrogen) treated, e.g. 200 mg testosterone subcutaneously

 (v) strange mare or gelding

6.3   Teasing technique

The object is to confront each mare individually with the teaser. The problem is that this is labour intensive and can be hazardous to personnel (foals also require restraint).

• ideally mares are teased at a board (teaser one side, mare the other) for at least 5 minutes. The initial reaction of the mare may be misleading; requires 2−3 people

• the teaser may be in a small enclosure, part of the side of which is a teasing board (with rail over to prevent teaser escaping). Mares are brought up to the board individually with the teaser unrestrained. Teaser may become difficult to handle; requires 1−2 people

• the teaser may be used in his own box in the same way, but the box door soon becomes damaged

• the teaser, usually a pony, is walked through a field of mares and individuals are approached. There is some danger to the teaser and handler and teasing is not as thorough; requires 1 or 2 persons

• taking the teaser to fence or gate; relies on mares approaching the teaser. Many mares will be 'missed' therefore this method is not recommended

• playing audio-tapes of stallion's calls.

6.4   Restraint of the mare for covering

Ideally this should be minimal but since the stallion is usually more valuable and vulnerable than the mare, some restraint is usually used.

• for a quiet mare, known to be 'well in season', a head collar or bridle are sufficient

• twitch is usually sufficient for a slightly nervous mare, or one 'going off'. It is essential for a mare of unknown temperament. It is easier if the mare is to stand in a preselected position, e.g. in a hollow to allow covering by a smaller stallion. Use twitch with a short handle which clips on to the head collar, or a very long handle so that holder can stand well clear of fore-limbs

• felt or canvas/leather boots help take the sting out of the kick.

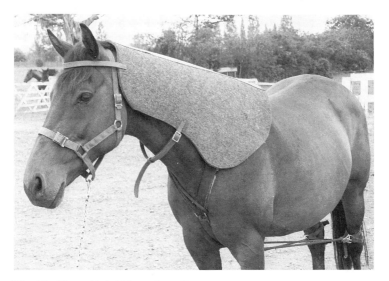

Fig. 6.1. Mare with hobbles and a collar.

They are slightly hazardous to apply and remove. The mare often 'dances' due to unfamiliar sensation and may kick until they come off. Often comes off if the mare moves frequently
• hobbles with side lines almost completely prevent mare from kicking (Fig. 6.1) but:
1 they are hazardous to apply to a difficult mare;
2 they must have quick release mechanism on mare's chest in case mare and/or stallion become entangled
• lifting left fore-leg with rope or special leather leg strap with quick release mechanism — release when stallion has mounted or if the mare stumbles. This method is useful for maiden mare that tries to run forward or buck
• tranquilizers — not recommended as mare may fall
• stallions' instinct. Some stallions take measures to avoid being kicked:
  (i) mounting the mare from side or quarters and then swivel round to right position. Stallion may get both feet over mare's back and be forced to dismount
  (ii) biting the mare's lower left leg just before mounting — she lifts the leg and is off balance
  (iii) nudging the mare's left hip with right shoulder just before mounting — the mare is off balance

• bandaging the mare's tail helps to prevent hairs from being introduced into the vulva and allows the stallion handler to observe the position of the horse's penis

NB, do not clean the mare's vulva with antiseptic. If necessary remove gross contamination with water and dry well.

6.5   Injuries during covering

Stallion

Usually traumatic due to:

• kicks on the penis or back leg (stifle joint)
• haematoma in the corpus cavernosum of the penis due to the mare twisting sideways suddenly during covering
• stallion slipping and falling
• any injury to the penis usually causes prolapse and swelling (haematoma and oedema). Treatment is conservative, i.e. cold water, support for the penis and protection from excoriation. Do not give tranquilizers
• inguinal or scrotal hernia can occur during covering
• laceration to the dorsum of the penis due to sutures in the mare's vulva
• psychological damage, particularly to young horses, due to a rough handler or mare
• fatal haemorrhage, due to rupture of the aorta, occurs rarely.

Mare

Bites

• most stallions nip the mare's buttocks, flanks and legs before mounting. Some stallions bite the mare's neck during covering
• bites at the rear end rarely cause trouble but occasionally a stallion appears to dislike a mare, and bites her savagely without mounting
• excessive checking of the stallion may cause loss of erection and disinclination to mount
• drenching the mare's hindquarters in urine from another mare in heat may induce the stallion to cover the mare normally
• stallion may cause obvious trauma to mare's neck; this is avoided by:
 (i) placing a stick between the stallion's teeth when he tries to bite
 (ii) covering the mare's neck with a sack, cloth or a leather collar

Vaginal trauma

Clinical signs are haemorrhage and straining due to:

 (i) rupture of hymen remnants in maidens (12.15)

 (ii) rupture of vagina — usually dorsal or lateral fornix and retro-peritoneal. If rupture is diagnosed, give parenteral antibiotic cover

 (iii) cervical damage and rupture of the uterus are rare

• some stallions commonly cause vaginal trauma due to either large penis or dorsal thrusting.

• trauma can be avoided by inserting a padded cylinder (breeder's roll) between the stallion's abdomen and the mare's rump during coitus, i.e. this reduces the length of the penis in the vagina.

7 / Normal pregnancy

7.1   Uterine changes

• the uterus becomes progressively more turgid, tubular (tonic) and more narrow from about 15 days to 21 days post-ovulation
• by 21 days the uterine body and horns feel sausage or hose-pipe like due to tone, but:
1   tone may not be marked in older parous mares or maiden mares
2   post-partum involution may produce turgidity similar to the tone of pregnancy
3   acute endometritis causes turgidity similar to pregnancy
4   the uterus is tonic in some cases of prolonged dioestrus
• at about 21 days a swelling develops at the base of one of the uterine horns. This part of the uterus houses the conceptus and is 1.5−3 cm in diameter; the swelling bulges ventrally
• the uterine wall over the conceptus is thin, but the persistent

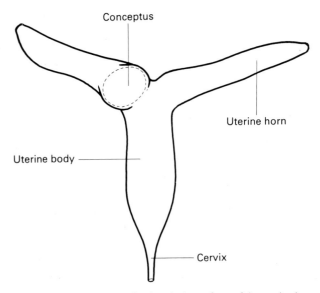

Fig. 7.1. The conceptus becomes fixed at the base of one of the uterine horns on the 16th day after ovulation.

tone in the adjacent uterus keeps conceptus in place after day 16 (Fig. 7.1)

• as the conceptus grows the swelling becomes larger but remains roughly spherical. The distal part of the pregnant horn remains tonic

• by 60 days the swelling is about 12 cm in diameter and fills the pregnant horn. The body and non-pregnant horn are still tonic

• after 60 days the swelling usually becomes less tense and starts to involve the body and non-pregnant horn

• by 90 days the whole uterus is filled with fluid (**8.3**)

• further distension of the uterus causes the ventral surface of the uterine body to lie against the ventral body wall. The dorsal surface of the uterus is suspended by the broad ligaments

• distinction between body and horns becomes less obvious

• at day 36 endometrial cups start to develop in a ring round the equator of the conceptus

• cups produce equine chorionic gonadotrophin (eCG) or PMSG

• as the conceptus becomes larger, cups are adjacent to its dorsal aspect

• NB, cups are not palpable per rectum

• at 100−150 days the cups become necrotic and slough off the surface of the endometrium, and come to lie between that and the allantochorion

• invaginations develop in the allantochorion to accommodate the dead cup tissue — these become chorio-allantoic pouches or vesicles (Fig. 7.2).

7.2   Development of the conceptus

• sufficient sperms for fertilization are present in the fallopian (uterine) tube by 4−6 hours after coitus

• the ovum is fertilized in the uterine tube to produce conceptus

• conceptus reaches the uterus about 5 days after ovulation

• non-fertilized ova remain in the uterine tube and degenerate

• the conceptus is mobile in the uterine horns and body for up to 16 days

• it then becomes lodged at the base of one of the horns, usually the narrower one (not related to the side of ovulation)

• the embryo develops in ventral wall of conceptus and is free of the trophoblast wall by 20 days

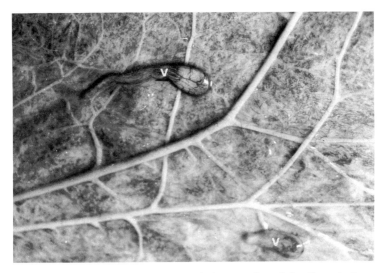

Fig. 7.2. Chorio-allantoic vesicles (v) on the inner surface of the allantochorion.

• development of early allantois between embryo and trophoblast pushes the embryo dorsally (Fig. 7.3)
• as the yolk sac (which is dorsal to the embryo) becomes smaller and the conceptus becomes larger, the embryo travels further dorsally
• the mesoderm surrounding the yolk sac carries blood vessels
• the umbilicus will be attached dorsally (at the base of one uterine horn).
• after about 35 days, most organogenesis is completed and the embryo is called a fetus.
• the fetus remains in the pregnant horns until about 70−80 days, but is then usually in the body until 6−7 months
• by now the fetus is becoming too big to remain only in the body, and its hind quarters begin to occupy one horn, usually the original pregnant horn
• after this time the fetus cannot change its presentation
• until just before second stage labour, the fetus is usually in a ventral or lateral position with limbs, head and neck flexed.

7.3   Placenta and fetal membranes

Placenta
The placenta of the mare is epitheliochoriol (no loss of maternal

tissue) and diffuse (throughout the whole uterus, except at the cervix and the uterine ends of the Fallopian tube).
• villi of trophoblast from the chorion occupy crypts in micro-cotyledons of the endometrium
• attachment begins around 25 days and becomes more extensive as the allantochorion comes to fill more of the uterine luteum
• physical attachment of the placenta is not strong, as diffuse placentation allows adequate surface area for physiological function
• physical stability of the placenta is aided by:
(i) Tone of uterus adjacent to conceptus in early stages.
(ii) large volume of fluid keeping whole of uterus distended in later stages.
• weak physical attachment of the placenta ensures easy separation of allanto-chorion from the endometrium in third stage labour (**9.6**).

Fetal membranes
Fetal membranes consist of:
• *allanto-chorion*, or *chorio-allantoic membrane* (CAM). The outer surface of this membrane (chorion) is covered with micro-villi which are composed of capillaries and a little stromal tissue and an epithelium. This surface looks velvet-like and red. The inner surface is shiny, and through it can be seen the larger veins and arteries which emanate from the umbilical vessels
• *amnion*, which is formed by fusion of the allantois and amnion proper (this membrane would more correctly be called allanto-amnion). It is a white membrane containing many tortuous blood vessels (these become straighter as pregnancy progresses)
• the amnion and CAM are completely separate from each other, and only attached indirectly via the umbilical cord
• the cord traverses the allantoic cavity, and at the level of the amnion, the two veins join to form one vessel in the amniotic cavity
• the amniotic part of the cord also contains the urachus, a canal which conducts fetal urine from the bladder to the allantoic cavity
• the amniotic cord, and inner surface of the amnion, are often covered with small rough plaques of cells which contain glycogen
• twisting of the umbilical cord and/or dilations of the urachus are often associated with abortion (**18.4**)
• *the hippomanes* is a soft calculus of cellular and inorganic debris which forms in the allantoic cavity. Occasionally there are accessory

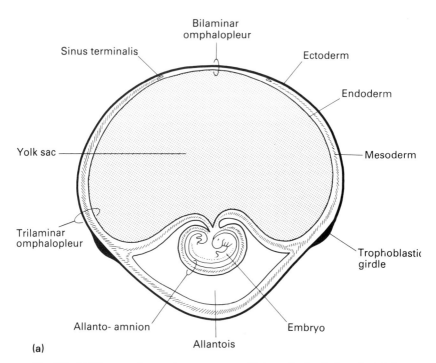

Fig. 7.3. (a) Diagram of an equine conceptus at 30 days; the developing allantois is pushing the embryo dorsally and the vascular mesoderm is enveloping the yolk sac. (b) Diagram of part of the equine conceptus at 55 days; the yolk sac is becoming vestigal and will be enveloped by the blood vessels of the umbilical cord.

small hippomanes either free in the fluid or attached to the CAM particularly on the chorio-allantoic pouches (wrongly called 'false hippomanes').

7.4   Endocrine changes

The major hormonal events during gestation are:
1   Progesterone concentrations (from the CL verum) usually fall slightly at 14−16 days post-ovulation, but are rarely less than 1 ng/ml plasma. They may also fall again around the 30th−40th day. Thereafter values rise due to:
• stimulation of greater progesterone out-put from the CL verum by eCG (PMSG)

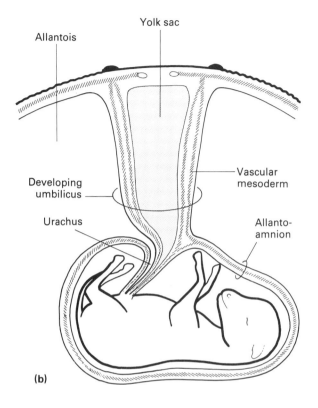

(b)

- ovulation and lutenization of follicles forming secondary progesterone producing CLs

Progesterone thereafter is also produced by the placenta (both fetal and maternal components), so that when the CLs regress at about 120 days, pregnancy is maintained by placental progesterone

- placental progesterone acts locally, so blood concentrations are low after 5 months
- progesterone values in blood rise just before parturition.

2 LH concentrations are low throughout gestation

3 FSH is released episodically up to 40 days and probably also to about 100 days.

- before 40 days it is responsible for follicular development, and thereafter is probably synergistic with eCG in causing marked ovarian activity.

4 Oestrogens. Until 100 days circulating oestrogen values are low; thereafter the fetal gonads and placenta produce vast quantities of equilin, equilenin, oestrone and $17-\beta$ oestradiol.

• both blood and urine concentrations of these oestrogens remain high until 300 days, after which they decline to term

• oestrone is conjugated to oestrone sulphate in the fetal liver; the amount of this hormone in the maternal circulation is an indication of fetal 'wellbeing'

5 Equine chorionic gonadotrophin (eCG) or PMSG is produced by the endometrial cups and appears in the circulation at about day 40. Values rise rapidly to peak at $60-70$ days and thereafter decline.

• there is marked individual variation in the amount and length of time for which eCG is produced, e.g. it may disappear by 60 days or still be present at 150 days

7.5 Cervical changes

• in early pregnancy the cervix is identical to dioestrus (**4.6**) but at speculum examination may be deflected up, down or laterally. This is because the cervix is stuck to the vaginal wall by mucus.

• as pregnancy progresses, the anterior vagina and external os of the cervix become covered in very tacky, dry mucus.

• after the fifth month the cervix becomes softer and shorter possibly due to high concentrations of circulating oestrogens.

• NB, a finger can be passed along the cervical canal at all stages of pregnancy. This is undesirable as pregnancy failure follows due to introduction of infection and (in later pregnancy) rupture of the allantochorion.

7.6 Ovarian changes

• primary corpus luteum (CL) of pregnancy (*corpus luteum verum*) is not lysed at 14 days and persists until $120-150$ days

• $18-40$ days; ovaries are characterized by presence of many (up to 3 cm diameter) follicles. Ovulations are uncommon

• $40-120$ days; extensive ovarian activity with multi-follicular development, ovulations and luteinization of unruptured follicles. Secondary corpora lutea are formed

• 120 days—term; follicular activity ceases, all corpora lutea regress and ovaries become small and inactive

• position of ovaries up to 2 months is as for the non-pregnant mare. Thereafter they are pulled anteriorly and medially but remain dorsal to the uterus. Tension on the utero-ovarian ligaments makes the ovaries less mobile. Not usually palpable after 5 months because they are difficult to reach.

7.7   Twinning (18.3, 20.2)

• twin pregnancy is undesirable in the mare as it often terminates in abortion of both fetuses or birth of dead or under-nourished foals at term
• equine twins are dizygotic, i.e. from two ova. In about two-thirds of cases they develop one in each horn, in the others two conceptuses are adjacent at the base of the same horn; the latter situation is most common in foaling mares
• in many cases early death of one embryo and subsequent resorption allows the other conceptus to develop normally
• conceptuses that both develop past 60 days compete for placental space, resulting in:
 (i) early death of one small conceptus trapped at the tip of the uterine horn. May be evidence of this when the other (normal) foal is born at term (but fetal 'moles' are yolk sac anomalies, not twins).
 (ii) death of one fetus later, followed by continuation of pregnancy and production of an undernourished live foal near or after term with a fetal 'mummy'.
 (iii) death of one fetus later, followed by abortion of both fetuses, one usually alive. This occurs when the viable pregnancy can't produce enough progesterone to maintain pregnancy.
• diagnosis of twin pregnancy (20.2)
• management of twin pregnancy (20.1, 20.3)
• NB, udder development and milk production during gestation often denotes (a) death of a twin and may be followed by abortion or survival of the other fetus, (b) placental separation due to other causes.

7.8   Duration of pregnancy

• pregnancy length is of the order of 330−345 days in the mare, but is very variable, with extremes of 310−370 days or even longer occurring not infrequently.

• factors which affect pregnancy length are:

(i) date of conception; mares which conceive (and therefore foal) early in the year have long gestation lengths, probably because maximal growth of the foal occurs when natural food (grass) is not available and nutrition may be poor.

(ii) sex of foal; male foals have gestation lengths about 1 day longer than females on average.

(iii) individual variation; some mares have similar gestation lengths in successive pregnancies, others do not.

(iv) placental lesions may cause retardation of the growth of the fetus and an extension in pregnancy length. The foal may still be dysmature at birth.

(v) death of one twin and continuation of pregnancy may result as (iv).

• problems associated with pregnancies which exceed expected duration are (**9.3**):

(i) mainly owner orientated, e.g. owner sat up or took time off work, etc. for expected foaling which did not materialize.

(ii) foal may be oversized and cause dystocia — this is rare. Most long pregnancies are essential to ensure that the foal is mature at birth, and dysmature foals may be produced after a normal length pregnancy.

(iii) foal may be dead and mummifying or putrifying, etc; unfounded fear as death of a single fetus invariably results in rapid abortion (**17.3, 17.4**).

• NB, mares will foal when they are ready, not necessarily when they are calculated to be 'due'.

8 / Pregnancy diagnosis

8.1   Absence of subsequent oestrus

This method is commonly (unwittingly) used by stud personnel and owners as an initial screening method, but:
• some mares show oestrus when pregnant, and may be covered, especially if restrained: this rarely causes embryonic death, unless the cervix is opened during coitus — more likely in old or recently foaled mares.
• it is commonly assumed that the mare will be in oestrus 21 days after covering (**2.1**). Teasing may therefore be too late in either normal or short cycles.
• if the mare returns home after covering the owners may not be able to recognize oestrus.
• some mares which return to oestrus after covering may show no signs, especially those with foals (silent heat—**12.4**).
• non-pregnant mares may not return to heat, usually due to prolonged dioestrus (**4.8**) and occasionally due to anoestrus (lactational or at the end of the season or during periods of inclement weather, especially in mares foaling in January and February—**4.1**).

8.2   Progesterone concentrations

Progesterone concentrations in plasma (or milk) can be measured by:
1   *Radio-immunoassay*; sample must be sent (delivered) to laboratory and result may take two or more days to obtain.
2   *Eliza tests*; these can be conducted in a practice laboratory and results are rapid (horse plasma can be harvested in 30 minutes without a centrifuge). Cost per sample is lowest where many are assayed (standards do not need repeating).
• At 18−20 days post-ovulation pregnant mares should have plasma progesterone concentration above 1 ng/ml
BUT
• not all mares with high progesterone are pregnant (cf, prolonged dioestrus, early fetal death and mares with short cycles)
• mis-timing of sampling (relative to previous ovulation) will give erroneous result

- occasionally pregnant mares have low progesterone
- thorough clinical examination gives cheaper and more complete and accurate information on the mare's reproductive status.

8.3   Clinical examination

- ovarian palpation contributes little to pregnancy diagnosis as large follicles may be present and the CL is not palpable
- uterine and cervical changes are described in **7.1** and **7.5**
- at 18−21 days; good uterine tone and a tightly closed cervix (as assessed *per rectum* or *vaginam*) are indicators of pregnancy
- 21−60 days; good uterine tone, swelling at the base of one or both (twins) uterine horns and tightly closed cervix. All must be present for positive diagnosis
- 60−120 days; swelling becomes less discrete, horns become more difficult to palpate and body becomes more fluid filled and prominent. May be intrapelvic and tense in young mares. Can be difficult time for diagnosis. Continuity with the cervix helps identification of the uterus. Fetus sometimes balloted (**7.1, 7.2**)
- 120 days to term; cervix becomes softer, fetus becomes more obvious. Dorsal surface of uterine body always in reach. Fetus often felt moving after 6 months
- *optimum time for rectal examination* depends on:
  (i) experience of clinician — later examinations (up to 60 days) are usually easiest.
  (ii) time of year — the later the examination the more time is lost if the mare is not pregnant.
  (iii) value of mare — early positive examinations should be repeated to detect pregnancy failure. Repeat examinations are recommended up to 40 days. After this pregnancy failure is rarely followed by fertile oestrus (**17.5**).

8.4   Ultrasound scanning (3.5)

- real time ultrasound scanners are now established in equine stud practice for the diagnosis of early pregnancy, and the recognition and early management of twin pregnancies
- with experience, these machines will undoubtedly also be used for assessing other facets of reproduction in mares, e.g. recognition of corpus haemorrhagicum, uterine abnormalities, etc.

- most machines currently in use are linear, i.e. emit a parallel beam of ultrasound which produces a rectangular picture
- scanners are no substitute for clinical acumen, as correct positioning of the scanner is necessary for accurate interpretation of results
- basically and simply, ultrasound is reflected as it passes through tissue. Dense tissue reflects most of the ultrasound which reaches it and appears white on conventional machines. Liquid reflects no sound and appears black. Soft tissue organs reflect varying degrees of sound and show up as different shades of grey
- for pregnancy diagnosis, the non-reflective (non-echogenic) fetal fluid is the earliest evidence of gestation, but later the reflective (echogenic) embryo and fetus can be seen. Within this the first embryonic organ to be recognized is the heart (non-echogenic and pulsating)
- various landmarks in the development of the pregnancy which can be identified by ultrasound are shown in Fig. 8.1

N B
- the complete uterus (both horns and body) must be scanned to diagnose twin pregnancy (**20.2**)
- twins in the same horn can be difficult to diagnose until two embryos (after about 25 days) can be identified
- early pregnancies can be confused with ovarian follicles and cysts in the uterine lumen or endometrium.

8.5 Equine chorionic gonadotrophin

(eCG, PMSG) appears in the blood in detectable levels about 40 days after ovulation and usually persists for 60−100 days. The hormone is produced by the endometrial cups (**7.4**).

The amount of eCG produced varies greatly from mare to mare, and mares carrying twins do not necessarily produce more than those with singleton pregnancies.

- errors in the test are due to:
 (i) sampling at the wrong time.
 (ii) the mare producing little eCG after 60 days.
 (iii) mares in which pregnancy fails after the endometrial cups form continue to produce eCG (false positive) (**17.5**).
 (iv) Samples not tested immediately may lose potency.
- eCG tested for by radio-immunoassay (commercial laboratories), haemagglutination-inhibition test (commercial laboratories and

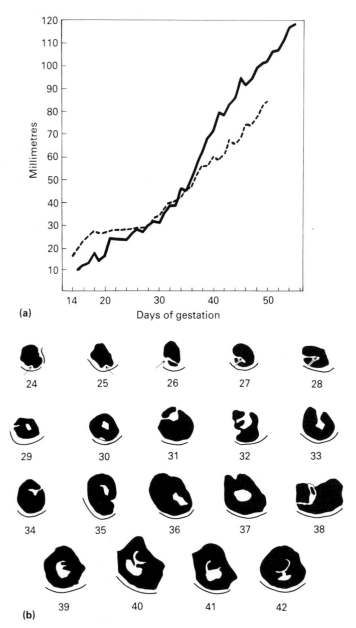

Fig. 8.1. (a) Mean diameter of the conceptual swelling as measured by ultrasound
(------) and as assessed by palpation (——). (b) Daily development of echogenic
structures within the conceptus between days 24 and 42. The embryo is first seen
ventrally on day 21 and appears to move dorsally as development continues. The
embryo is indicated by an arrow for days 24 to 28. (Reproduced from Allen W. E. &
Goddard P. J. (1984) Equine Veterinary Journal **16**, 509–14, by permission of the
Editor.)

test kit for practitioners), and latex agglutination test (test kit for practitioners).

8.6 Placental oestrogens

These reach peak levels in plasma and urine at 150 days, and concentrations remain high until after 300 days. The amount of oestrogen produced is so great that false positives do not occur due to other conditions. False negative results are also very rare after 150 days. Oestrogens are tested for in the urine — free oestrogens produce a colour reaction with sulphuric acid. The Cuboni test is the most accurate but involves extraction procedure using benzene (carcinogen) and acid. The Lunaas test is simpler, uses acids but is sometimes difficult to interpret.

Plasma. Assays for oestrone sulphate are being evaluated.

9 / Normal parturition

9.1 Endocrine control

• parturition is rapid in the mare and the endocrine control is poorly understood
• unlike other species, parturition is preceded by a decrease in circulating oestrogen concentrations and an increase in progesterone
• prostaglandins, oxytocin, corticosteroids and relaxin are probably involved in the initiation of parturition
• the role of prolactin is unknown; placental lactogen is not found in the horse.

9.2 Preparation of the environment

1 Mares probably foal most naturally outside, but:
• constant surveillance is difficult
• other horses may molest the foal
• fetal membranes may be predated before inspection
• foal may be damaged in wire and hedges, or drown in ponds and ditches, etc.
2 Mares foaling in boxes require:
• adequate room — at least 12' × 12'
• minimal disturbance
• good bedding — well compacted over concrete floor and built up at the walls
• minimal low-level feed bins; water bucket should be off the floor
• lots of time and patience

9.3 The 'overdue' foal (7.8)

1 The biggest problem the foaling mare has is her owner, because:
• the owner expects foaling to occur 11 months after conception — gestation length is very variable
• the owner does not understand that the mare will foal when she is ready, not when the owner thinks she is 'due'
• the owner has taken time off work to stay up at night to observe the foaling. He/she is now exhausted, must return to work and worry about the 'expectant mother'

- the owner suspects that an 'overdue' mare is harbouring a dead foal — mares do not retain dead (single) foals; they are aborted
- the owner thinks the foal will be oversized if pregnancy is long — this is very unlikely as long pregnancies usually indicate slow growth of the foal; fetal oversize is rare in horses, irrespective of parent size
- the owner has planned a party to coincide with foaling — mares need minimal disturbance during parturition, and interference can cause the mare to delay expulsion and might result in dystocia
- celebrate nothing until the foal is a week old!

2 In the event of a mare not foaling at the expected time, the veterinary surgeon may:

- examine the mare *per rectum* to confirm that she is pregnant
- confirm, by feeling fetal movement, that the foal is alive (to reassure the owner)
- confirm, if palpation of the foal's head is possible, that it is in an anterior presentation
- possibly, examine the cervix *per vaginam* for evidence of relaxation and liquification of cervical mucus — the cervix in late pregnancy is normally very soft, the canal is only $\frac{1}{2}-1$ cm long. The fetus is often palpable *per vaginam*.
- Pre-partum the cervical mucus is very tacky — repeated examinations are not recommended
- check that the expected foaling date has been calculated correctly

9.4 First stage labour

- the beginning of first stage cannot be recognized
- this is the preparation for the expulsive (second) stage
- the mare is restless, looks at her flanks and shifts her weight from one hind limb to another — these signs can be seen for months before foaling
- slackening of the sacro-sciatic ligaments and relaxation of the vulva are inconsistent signs
- the escape of a honey-like precursor of colostrum (wax), onto the ends of the teats is a good sign that the mare is in the 'first stage' — but some mares expel obvious milk for days before foaling and others never wax-up
- there is a rise in the calcium and potassium content of udder secretion before foaling, and a fall in sodium; the concentrations of

potassium and sodium become similar (about 40 mmol/litre) 24−48 hours pre-partum

• the signs of first stage labour are basically those exhibited by a mare suffering myometrial contractions prior to opening of the cervix — the intensity of the signs depend on the mare and her environment

• mares in first stage labour may hold their breath and grunt, but they do not normally strain — this is explosive and expulsive and occurs during second stage.

9.5   Second stage labour, i.e. expulsion (see also Chapter 24)

• the cervix opens relatively quickly to allow the separating CAM to bulge into the vagina (7.3)

• eventually the pressure in the vagina causes either the CAM to rupture, with the visible loss of allantoic fluid from the vulva, or the mare to strain

• either event marks the beginning of second stage labour and has evoked Ferguson's reflex, i.e. vaginal distension causes oxytocin release and further myometrial contractions; if the CAM hasn't ruptured, it does so now

• mare is usually in lateral recumbency

• straining involves tensing of abdominal muscles and rigidity of all four limbs

• the amnion, a white glistening membrane, soon becomes visible at the vulva containing fluid and/or a fetal foot

• both front feet (one further forward than the other) and the nose should appear in quick succession

• after expulsion of the head the mare often stands and eats, or may roll to change the position of the foal

• further straining ensures delivery of the chest and hips

• if left undisturbed, the mare may lie for some time with the foal's hind limbs in her vagina

• the foal is born in the amnion, but ruptures this when it attempts to sit up

• movement of the dam or foal causes the umbilical cord to rupture close to the abdominal wall

• the mare's instinct is to lick the foal dry, but not to eat the membranes

• second stage labour usually occurs at night, and lasts 5−25 (mean 15) minutes.

9.6 Third stage labour (expulsion of the membranes)

• has usually occurred within three hours.
• mare may show signs of abdominal pain due to continued uterine contractions.
• the weight of the amnion gently pulling on the CAM via the umbilical cord causes separation.
• the CAM is turned inside out during expulsion (Fig. 9.1).
• the membranes should be kept and inspected to ensure that they are complete (**21.3**).

9.7 Induction of parturition

Indications
• rarely necessary because long pregnancies are physiological and fetal oversize is not a problem
• useful in a very uncomfortable mare running milk with ventral oedema and relaxation of the cervix.

Criteria for induction
• adequate gestation length, i.e. in excess of 320 days although most veterinary surgeons will not consider induction until well past this time
• adequate mammary development, preferably with milk
• may give oestradiol, e.g. 5−10 mg 24 hours previously to relax cervix.

Drugs used
• prostaglandins at twice the luteolytic dose
• oxytocin 40−60 iu intramuscularly
• oxytocin 6 iu intravenously.

Expected outcome
• parturition may proceed normally within 1½ hours
• initially, especially after oxytocin, the mare may be very uncomfortable and sweat profusely; this may be followed by a calm period before second stage labour

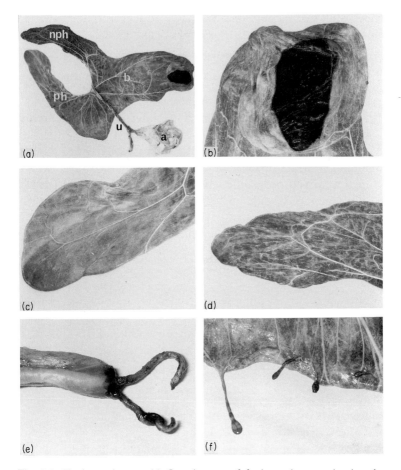

Fig. 9.1. Fetal membranes. (a) Complete set of fetal membrances showing the amnion **a**, umbilical cord **u** and the inner surface of the chorio-allantois **b** body; **ph**, pregnant horn; **nph**, non-pregnant horn. (b) Site where the allantochorion ruptured at the cervix. (c) Tip of pregnant horn (oedematous). (d) Tip of non-pregnant horn. (e) End of umbilical cord showing the umbilical arteries which ruptured within the foal's abdomen. (f) Chorio-allantoic vesicles containing the remnants of the endometrial cups.

- progress should be monitored by palpation of the cervix *per vaginam*
- repeat doses of either drug may be necessary
- expulsion of the foal may require assistance
- parturition may not be induced in some mares

• retrospectively, mares that foal most rapidly after induction are mares which were closest to their physiological foaling time.

Complications
• Veterinary Surgeon should remain close at hand once induction has started although this may be expensive
• dystocia may occur due to inability or unwillingness of the foal to rotate during expulsion; this may be a sign of unreadiness for birth
• the foal may be produced dead (suffocated) in the chorio-allantoic membrane.
• immature and dysmature foals have trouble adapting to extra-uterine life and may die.

10 / Post-partum events

10.1 Uterine involution

- amazingly rapid after normal parturition
- histologically there is no disruption of the endometrium
- the uterine horn which housed the fetus will remain larger
- difficult to define when involution is complete, i. e. when the previously pregnant horn is no longer identifiable by palpation
- the uterine cervix remains relaxed until after the foal heat ovulation
- new pregnancies almost invariably establish in the smaller uterine horn
- tone of involution after foal heat makes early manual diagnosis of pregnancy more difficult — enlargement at the base of previously pregnant horn may be mistaken for an 18−28 day conception.

10.2 Post-partum infection

- bacteria enter many mares' uteri post-partum
- this can be reduced by immediately suturing or clipping the dorsal vulva after delivery
- post-partum uterine flora is usually dominated initially by coliforms, and later by β-haemolytic streptococci
- post-partum colonization of the uterus by bacteria is a normal event
- after normal parturition, most mares eliminate bacteria before the foal heat
- very little discharge is normally seen from the vulva after the first few days post-partum.

10.3 The foal heat

- usually starts 5−9 days post-partum
- may not occur in mares that foal very early in the year or in adverse climatic conditions of seasonal anoestrus
- foal often develops a physiological scour at this heat, which makes identification in the mare more obvious
- occasionally the mare is reluctant to show signs of oestrus due to

maternal instinct (i.e. silent heat); this is more likely to occur during subsequent heats

• silent heat in this instance should be prevented by either holding the foal securely at mare's head, or confining it to a loose box out of earshot; the mare may need to be twitched

• opinion as to whether the foal heat should be used or not is divided; each mare should be evaluated individually according to the following criteria:

  (i) Don't use foal heat if:

    involution is physically poor

    mare has discharge or positive culture (or neutrophils) at covering time (**14.3**)

    mare had dystocia or retained fetal membranes (**21.3**)

    mare foaled early and an even earlier foal is not required

    if the mare has ovulated by the eight day post-partum she is unlikely to conceive.

 (ii) Do use foal heat if:

    mare foaled late in season

    post-partum events seem normal

    involution is adequate

    mare is known to have aberrent cycles after the foal heat.

(iii) Advantages of using the foal heat:

    easily recognizable because of foal scour and record of recent foaling

    avoids the confusion of erratic cyclic behaviour thereafter

    may be last chance of conception for late foalers.

(iv) Disadvantages of using foal heat:

    conception rate is lower than for other heats

    subsequent pregnancy loss may be higher

    covering a mare with a diseased endometrium may prejudice against conception at a later heat or even cause permanent damage, especially after the first foal.

11 / Normal expectations of fertility

11.1 Conception and foaling rates

- horses have always been selected for ability or conformation, i.e. they have never been selected for fertility
- consequently horses are relatively infertile when compared with other domesticated species because:
- (i) seminal quality is very variable between stallions and
- (ii) many mares exhibit erratic and unpredictable reproductive behaviour.
- conception rates at any one heat are about 40−50% in large breeds of horse; ponies tend to do better
- some apparently normal mares require covering at up to 4 heats to become pregnant; others fail to conceive until the next season
- overall conception rates at the end of the season vary between 50% and 90%, and this depends on:
- (i) fertility of the stallion
- (ii) fertility of the mares
- (iii) value of the horses involved, i.e. constant veterinary attention to mares where cost warrants this, results in better fertility *and* very expensive stallions do not usually attract mares which are difficult to settle.
- pregnancy loss, after confirmed conception is about 15%, again this figure is lowest for ponies (**17.2**, **17.4**)
- for the Hunter Improvement Scheme stallions, only 60% of mares produce a foal the next year, i.e. at least 40% of mare-owners are disappointed
- horse breeding at any level is a gamble because you may not get a foal, or the foal you do get may not be the one you want.

11.2 Effect of management on fertility

- most stallion owners want maximal fertility for their horses because this is their best form of advertising
- running a stud is a compromise between the expectations of the mare owners, the quality of the mares, the money involved and the expected value of the foals

- good studs tease mares regularly and individually; this involves the employment of sufficient staff
- mare owners who want to present their mare when in heat must be aware that the mare may have fooled them and that recently travelled mares may not be relaxed enough to accept service
- many mares which arrive at stud said by their owners to be in heat are not
- mares fail to exhibit heat for many reasons (**12.1, 12.2, 12.4**); this may be the fault of management but is more often a problem of the mare
- the length of time for which a mare fails to show heat before veterinary advice is sought depends on the policy of the stud and the attitude of the owner
- such a decision should involve consideration of:
  (i) cost of veterinary treatment.
  (ii) cost of keeping a mare at stud.
  (iii) stage of breeding season.
- veterinary attention to a brood mare may be of benefit to three different factions:
  (i) the stud in general, e.g. swabbing for venereal diseases (**14.1**) and post-mortem examination of aborted fetuses and dead foals, i.e. identification of specific diseases allows measures to be taken to prevent spread.
  (ii) the mare owner, e.g. examinations and treatment of mares not seen in heat, pregnancy diagnosis, treatment of mares with endometritis (**13.2**), and examination of mares which repeatedly fail to hold to service.
  (iii) the stud owner, e.g. examination to ascertain the time of ovulation so that the mare only needs to be covered on a limited number of occasions; if the stallion has a lot of mares booked to him (i.e. is popular) this procedure is necessary to facilitate organization of an efficient covering programme.
- mistakes made by mare owners which contribute to poor fertility include:
  (i) presenting the mare for one day when she is thought to be in season.
  (ii) taking the mare home after covering and assuming that failure to observe subsequent heat is a reliable indicator of pregnancy.
  (iii) not allowing the stud owner to request reasonable veterinary attention to the mare.

(iv) presenting a mare to stud late in the breeding season on a whim or due to a leg injury which precludes other use.

11.3 Methods of investigating reproductive function in mares

- visual examination of the mare for general health, udder development and perineal conformation
- manual examination of the tract *per rectum* to assess reproductive status and diagnose pregnancy
- real-time ultrasound examination *per rectum* to diagnose pregnancy and examine for twins
- manual examination *per vaginam* to assess reproductive status and identify lesions
- speculum examination per vaginam to assess reproductive status and collect cervical/uterine swabs
- swabbing uterus (via speculum or manually) to provide material for bacteriological culture and cytological examination
- biopsy of the uterus to provide a prognosis for mare's future breeding potential
- endoscopic examination of the uterus to identify lesions
- swabs from clitoris to identify carriers of venereal disease
- blood sampling for hormone analysis to (a) confirm mare's reproductive status and (b) pregnancy diagnosis (blood test)
- blood sampling for chromosome analysis in mares which fail to mature sexually.

12 / Non-infectious infertility in mares

12.1 Prolonged dioestrus (4.8)

1 Caused by persistence of CL in absence of pregnancy.
- CL can persist for up to three or more months
- not related to early pregnancy loss, as it commonly occurs in mares which have never been covered
- can occur after 25% of ovulations, i.e. it is common
- CL is not palpable in ovaries, but follicles of various sizes develop
- rarely one of these follicles ovulates to form a secondary CL; usually large follicles remain static or slowly regress
- due to persistent progesterone stimulation from the CL, the uterus usually becomes firm and tubular (tonic)
- the cervix is typical of late dioestrus and early pregnancy.

2 Signs are failure to return to oestrus, especially during the breeding season, i.e. after an ovulation.

3 Treatment is prostaglandin administration, which causes luteolysis and a return to oestrus in 3–5 days (ovulation in 7–10 days).

4 One dose is usually sufficient but repeated doses may be needed because:
- some CLs require repeated prostaglandin stimulation
- mare may have had a dioestrus ovulation and the young CL (under 5 days) will not respond to prostaglandin
- may be large pre-ovulatory follicle in the ovary at the time of prostaglandin administration. The rapid decrease in progesterone after luteolysis allows quick ovulation without signs of oestrus and a new luteal phase begins; when a large follicle is palpated before prostaglandin administration, the mare should be teased daily thereafter and covered immediately she shows signs of heat. Some large follicles regress, however, and subsequent ovulation is from a new one; this can't be anticipated.

12.2 Erratic behaviour early in the season (4.2)

1 Caused by mare trying, but failing, to produce ovulatory follicles:
- sequential examination of the ovaries reveals waves of follicular development and regression

- single examinations can be confusing
- prognosis for time of ovulatory oestrus is difficult
- uterus is usually thin walled
- cervix varies between typically anoestrus to that of early oestrus

2   Signs are erratic oestrous behaviour of varied intensity, usually causing total confusion.

3   Treatment at this stage may be of little avail but should be along the following lines for avoidance (**5.1**):

- house and feed mare for at least 2 months before covering is expected. For mares to be covered from late April onwards this is not necessary
- subject the mare to 16 hours good light per day
- feed the progestagen allyl trenbolone in food daily for 14–16 days if the mare shows some follicular activity — heat should occur soon after withdrawal of the drug
- ensure that lighting and housing routines are continued after the mare has gone to stud
- there are no drugs yet available which will stimulate a mare in deep or shallow anoestrus to come into heat

12.3   Erratic post-partum behaviour (**10.3**)

1   Failure to show 'foal heat' is uncommon; failure to show heat thereafter is more likely.

- mares may be having silent heats (see later) or exhibiting a temporary true anoestrus, i.e. flacid tract and inactive ovaries (**4.1**)

2   Signs are failure to return to heat after foaling, or after the foal heat.

3   Treatment depends on cause:

- anoestrus mares may respond to a course of allyl trenbolone
- mares with silent heat are treated as below.

12.4   Silent heat

1   A mare that will either not show signs of heat or will not allow covering although rectal and vaginal examinations confirm that she is in oestrus and is going to ovulate:

- usually seen in maiden mares or mares with young foals at foot; however, even a mare which usually 'shows well' can occasionally be affected

• must be distinguished from prolonged dioestrus in which there is also follicular development (**4.3**, **4.8**).

2   A mare is difficult to cover when she is physiologically in oestrus:

• mare should be restrained as described in **6.4**
• foal may be held in front of mare or confined out of earshot
• artificial insemination, if permitted, may be the last resort.

12.5 Split oestrus

• mare fails to show heat for 1−2 days during the middle of an otherwise normal oestrus, i.e. follicle continues to develop and eventually ovulates
• rarely diagnosed as the initial cessation of oestrus is thought to indicate that ovulation has occurred
• if recognized, the mare may be treated as for silent heat or return of normal behaviour may be awaited.

12.6 Failure of CL formation after ovulation

• evidence for the occurence of this abnormality is scanty; if it does occur, it is most likely at the beginning and the end of the breeding season — haemorrhage may occur into an unruptured follicle with subsequent luteinizations.

12.7 Cystic ovaries do not occur in mares

• the term cystic ovaries implies the presence of large fluid filled structures which are either abnormal *per se*, or have developed in an abnormal manner
• such structures do occur in the ovaries of many animals, but *not* in the mare
• situations where 'cystic ovaries' are wrongly diagnosed in mares are:

(i) mare's ovaries are large compared with those of cows and practitioners unfamiliar with this may misinterpret the normal mare ovary.

(ii) during the transition from anoestrus to regular cyclic behaviour there may be many persistent follicles in the ovaries (**4.2**, **12.2**); these are morphologically normal.

(iii) during prolonged dioestrus there is continued ovarian follicular activity not associated with heat — the ovaries are morphologically normal (**4.8, 12.1**).

(iv) during early pregnancy there is massive and persistent ovarian activity (**7.6**); this also occurs in pseudopregnancy (**17.5; 19.3**).

• situations where cysts can be associated with mare ovaries (but *not* called cystic ovaries) are:

 (i) fossa cysts. These are found *post-mortem* in older mares, and are very small (1−5 mm). They probably occur due to developing CH enveloping a small amount of the fimbrial epithelium and dragging it into the ovary as the CL matures. Masses of cysts at the ovulation fossa could theoretically impede ovulation.

(ii) para-ovarian cysts. These are remnants of the Wolffian duct system and are found in the ovarian capsule, fimbria and meso-salpynx; they do not affect fertility.

12.8 Nymphomania

True nymphomania probably doesn't exist in mares, but conditions which mimic it are:

• persistent oestrus during early spring; this is physiological and can be treated by trying to induce ovulation with hCG if a large follicle is present, or feeding allyl trenbolone if many small follicles are present (**5.1, 5.3, 12.2**)

• mares which are bad tempered or otherwise difficult to handle during oestrus; ovariectomy gives good results, but the likely outcome of this treatment can be tested by feeding allyl trenbolone to abolish heat

• mares that are persistently vicious and difficult with other horses; they may squirt urine and 'show', especially when handled behind. These mares have normal ovaries and their problem is not sexual but psychological. Ovariectomy usually has no effect, but allyl trenbolone treatment can be tried as an indicator

• granulosa cell tumour (**12.9**).

12.9 Granulosa cell tumour

• this name is used to describe a family of histologically and endocrinologically different tumours (sex cord/stromal cell tumours) of the mare's ovary (other ovarian tumours are very rare)

• they can occur at any age, but usually affect young mares (5–9 years)
• only one ovary is involved
• depending on the hormones that the tumour produces, the mare may show persistent anoestrus, persistent oestrus or virilism (male like behaviour)
• diagnosis is by rectal examination of the ovary; this is large (8–30 cm diameter) spherical and hard, and the opposite ovary is usually small and inactive
• *NB* other ovarian conditions which may be confused with granulosa cell tumours are: large post-ovulation haematoma — this gradually becomes small over a period of weeks and the mare cycles normally; large active ovaries in spring, prolonged dioestrus, early pregnancy and pseudopregnancy type II — both ovaries are usually involved (**12.7**); teratoma — a very rare tumour of the ovary
• treatment is ovarohysterectomy
• opposite ovary may take up to one year to resume normal function, but mare should breed again

12.10 Chromosome abnormalities

Turner's syndrome
• uncommon chromosomal abnormality which renders the mare sterile (63, X 0)
• ovaries are very small and non-functional, and the uterus is very thin-walled and difficult to palpate
• blood tests on chromosomes confirm the diagnosis
• fillies out of training, even at 4 years, may have a quiescent reproductive tract, and need more time to mature (**2.3**).

Intersex
• foal is thought to be a filly until puberty at which time the clitoris enlarges and becomes phallus like, urination occurs in an upwards direction and the filly exhibits male like behaviour
• treatment is surgical removal of the gonads, which are usually testes and are intra-abdominal; surgery to the clitoris (phallus) may also be necessary with uncertain results.

Chromosome abnormalities in subfertile mares
• recent investigations have shown that some mares which are

difficult to get 'in foal' have a male chromosome complement
(64, X Y)
- these mares show no physical or behavioural changes.

12.11 Abnormalities of the uterine tubes

- this is very rare in mares, and when they do occur they are
unlikely to be diagnosed *ante-mortem*.

12.12 Uterine cysts

- may be one or more cysts in the endometrium or myometrium
- these can be diagnosed with ultrasound and they do not usually
affect fertility; they are often difficult to distinguish from an early
pregnancy until the absence of an embryo can be ascertained (± 25
days) — cysts are most common in older mares
- rarely there are multitudes of small cysts, i.e. cystic degeneration
of the endometrium
- this may be associated with mucometra (constant production of
mucus by the uterus)
- the prognosis for fertility is hopeless.

12.13 Partial dilation of the uterus

- a permanent dilation at the base of one or (rarely) both uterine
horns
- probably the result of repeated pregnancies, but histologically is
associated with lymphstasis in that area
- dilation is easiest to palpate when the mare is in oestrus, i.e.
uterus is oedematous
- may allow persistence of uterine secretions and semen after
covering, predisposing to endometritis (**13.2**)
- treatment is as for mares with poor uterine resistance (**15.2**).

12.14 Lesions of the cervix

1   Fibrosis of the cervix is often seen in older mares; sometimes in
old maiden mares.
- may be due to trauma at foaling in some mares
- cervix relaxes only slightly when mare is in oestrus

• after covering most of the ejaculate may remain in the vagina and be subsequently lost
• immediately after covering a tubular vaginal speculum is introduced and any remaining ejaculate is immediately inseminated into the uterus
• predisposes to endometritis as normal post-covering exudate cannot escape
• mares which conceive in this manner do not have trouble foaling
• severe constriction of the cervical canal may contribute to the development of pyometra (**15.3**).
2   Adhesions:
• can completely occlude the cervical canal
• usually form as a result of trauma (covering or foaling)
• can be broken down manually but usually recur — devices intended to remain in the canal to prevent this are not reliable
• can be corrected by constant digital breakdown whilst in season over several cycles
• surgical correction is rarely attempted
• prognosis for fertility is poor
• may contribute to the development of pyometra (**15.3**).

12.15 Persistent hymen

• manual vaginal examination of maiden mares often reveals hymen tissue at the vestibulo-vaginal junction; this breaks down easily with manual pressure
• occasionally the hymen is complete and at 2−3 years of age a glistening membrane is seen to bulge from the vulva when the filly lies down or urinates
• manual examination reveals abrupt occlusion of the vagina just anterior to the urethral opening
• the hymen can be very tough and is ruptured by introducing a guarded needle or blade. or retracting the hymen to the vulva with forceps and incising
• incision allows the escape of milky secretions which have accumulated anterior to the hymen; there may be some blood
• the small incision is easily expanded using a finger and hand
• rarely there are numerous strands of tissue between vestibule and cervical area; these require extensive blunt surgery.

12.16 Vaginal bleeding

• bleeding from the vulva after a potentially traumatic incident, i.e. covering or foaling, requires further investigation (**6.5, 22.4**)
• spontaneous vaginal bleeding in non-pregnant mares:

(i) this is usually more obvious in the morning, probably because blood has accumulated in the vestibule whilst the mare was resting overnight.

(ii) haemorrhage occurs from varicose vessels in the remnants of the hymen usually at the dorsal vestibulo-vaginal junction.

(iii) treatment is ligation of these vessels under local or general anaesthesia.

• spontaneous vaginal bleeding in the pregnant mare:

(i) rarely may be due to placental separation and signifies that foaling/abortion is imminent.

(ii) usually occurs in late gestation from lesions similar to those in the non-pregnant mare.

(iii) no treatment is necessary and bleeding ceases post-partum.

13 / Infectious infertility

13.1 General considerations

- infections of the mare's uterus are common, but inflammation is usually confined to the endometrium
- systemic illness is only associated with inflammation of the whole uterus, i.e. metritis; this is rare and only occurs post-partum
- a transient endometritis occurs after a mare is covered and after she foals; this is a normal reaction to the foreign protein and bacteria which enter the uterus at this time and is normally resolved within 24 hours of service and within 6 days of foaling
- this 'physiological' endometritis is confirmed by finding bacteria and inflammatory cells in the uterine lumen, but may not produce an obvious discharge
- persistence of endometrial infection occurs when:
 (i) the mare's resistance to normal genital bacteria is reduced.
 (ii) specific invasive venereal pathogens are present.
- endometritis causes infertility by:
 (i) providing an unsuitable uterine environment for development of the conceptus.
 (ii) causing premature lysis of the CL thus ensuring very early pregnancy failure — this is the important reason why 'dirty' mares fail to conceive and suggests that later pregnancy failures cannot be due to mares having endometritis at the time of covering.
 (iii) causing placentitis and possible bacteraemia or septicaemia of the fetus in late pregnancy; this stimulates abortion.

13.2 Non-specific infections

- the vestibular and clitoral area of the mare normally has a harmless and constantly fluctuating bacterial population; the stallion's penis is colonized by similar organisms.
- washing and disinfecting the genitalia before service can reduce the bacterial population but:
 (i) no treatment will completely sterilize either area.
 (ii) overuse of antiseptics is contraindicated because removal of the normal bacterial population allows resistant and potentially dangerous bacteria (especially *Pseudomonas sp.*) to proliferate.

• contamination of the mare's uterus, which is where most of the ejaculate is deposited, is physiological. The debris and bacteria derive from the stallion's penis and the mare's vestibule and vulva.
• elimination of these bacteria under normal circumstances is rapid (i.e. less than 24 hours) and effective, but two situations arise where this is not possible.

Pneumovagina (wind sucking) (15.5)
• faulty conformation of the vulva and/or vestibulo-vaginal constriction allows the mare to aspirate air into the vagina
• aspiration is persistent and the vagina may be contaminated from the adjacent rectum
• aspiration causes dessication of the vaginal mucosa and predisposes to bacterial infection; this spreads forward to the cervix and uterus and causes a chronic endometritis
• recognition of the condition may be easy if the mare makes an obvious noise whilst walking
• some mares are insidious windsuckers and may only do so when relaxed or whilst shifting weight from one hind leg to another in a box
• diagnosis can therefore be difficult, but the presence of froth (air and mucus) in the vagina is pathognomonic
• treatment is by Caslick's operation which results in fusion of the dorsal vulval labia, thus reducing the size of the orifice to prevent pneumovagina.

Factors which predispose to pneumovagina
1 Negative intravaginal pressure; air can only enter the vagina if pressure there is less than atmospheric. This pressure difference is usually greater in horses than ponies, and pneumovagina is uncommon in ponies.
2 Damage to the vestibulo-vaginal junction, usually caused by over stretching; this can allow pneumovagina even though vulval conformation is normal.
3 Abnormal vulval conformation; normally the vulva slopes slightly forward and most of the length of its opening is below the level of the floor of the pelvis (ischium).
   Abnormal conformations include:
• vertical vulva in maidens, where more than half the orifice is dorsal to the ischium; this causes pneumovagina in fillies in training

- horizontal vulva; due to ageing and weight loss (e. g. in winter) the anus sinks forward and pulls the vulva with it, so that part of the dorsal opening lies horizontally on the floor of the ischium. This not only predisposes to pneumovagina but allows gross contamination of the vestibule with faecal material
- tears of the vulval lips or scars which cause distortion (**22.1**)

4 Rectovaginal fistula (**22.2**) and perineal laceration (**22.3**).

Caslick's operation

1 Introduce antibiotic into the uterus as described later (**15.1, 15.2**).

2 Clean the vulva with clean water and dry.

3 Ascertain the level (ventally) to which the vulva must be sutured; ideally this should be to the level of the ischial arch, but if conformation is very poor, i.e. the vulva is pulled dramatically forward, a compromise which allows just sufficient room for coitus should be reached (for severe perineal malformations Pouret's operation should be considered).

4 Infiltrate the vulval lips with local anaesthetic after suitable restraint:
- start at the most ventral point and use a small (23 g 1″) needle (Fig. 13.1)
- proceed dorsally stepwise, ensuring that the dorsal commisure is well infiltrated
- repeat on the other side
- for mares previously operated on, infiltrate deeply.

5 Using rat-toothed forceps and curved scissors cut a strip of mucocutaneous junction from the ventral limit of the anaesthetized area to the dorsal commisure on both sides; ensure that the incision is complete dorsally and only remove mucosa. For mares that have been previously operated on, radical dissection may be necessary before healthy (bleeding) tissue is reached.

6 Suture one side of the vulva to the other using simple interrupted sutures or a locking pattern:
- suture material may be permanent or absorbable (e. g. dexon)
- time of suture removal is not critical but must occur before next foaling
- mares that require covering subsequently should be resutured immediately if ripping occurs; otherwise a deep mattress suture of

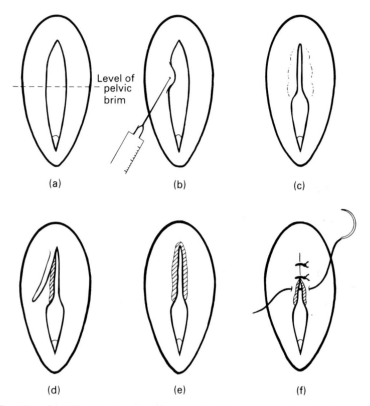

Fig. 13.1. Caslick's operation. (a) After restraining the mare, clean her vulva and ascertain the level of the floor of the pelvis. (b) Starting at this level, infiltrate the mucocutaneous junction of the vulva with local anaesthetic (10−20 ml) through a 21 g 1″ needle. (c) Infiltrate both sides up to the dorsal commisure. (d) Using rat toothed forceps and curved scissors cut a 2 mm strip of mucocutaneous junction from the anaesthetized area. (e) Ensure that tissue is removed completely from the dorsal commisure. (f) Coapt the cut areas with simple interupted sutures or a blanket stitch.

tape, after deep local infiltration, should be inserted before covering (breeders stitch)
- sutured mares must be 'opened' with scissors just before parturition; if not the vulva may tear laterally causing shortening and deformity of the vulva
- tears of the vulva should be attended to immediately post-partum (**21.1**); in this case local anaesthesia may not be necessary
- Pouret's operation is described in Fig. 13.2.

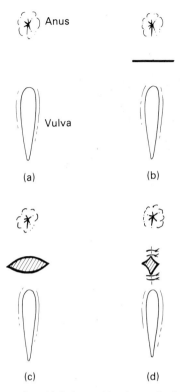

Fig. 13.2. Pouret's operation. (a) Induce epidural anaesthesia using about 10 ml of lignocaine (without adrenalin) in the sacro-coccygeal or first inter-coccygeal space. Clean the perineum. (b) Make a horizontal incision in the perineal body midway between the anus and vulva. (c) Bluntly dissect forward, without entering the rectum or vagina, to the retroperitoneal fat. Free the vagina laterally from its attachment to the pelvic wall. (d) Close the perineal skin converting the incision into a vertical one.

Reduced local uterine resistance

• some mares are unable to cope with the bacteria introduced during coitus; these mares develop a persistent post-coital endometritis which prevents conception

• the real reason for this problem is unknown, although it is suggested that there is a fault in the local immume response of the uterus

Diagnosis
Diagnosis (recognition) of the problem is hampered by:
• ignorance of the fact that the condition exists
• failure to recognize the significance of post-covering discharge; some discharge is accepted as normal and it is very difficult to decide when this might be pathological
• most mares are not observed closely during the 2 weeks following the end of heat; dioestrus discharge therefore often goes unobserved. Endometritis causes a shortening of the luteal phase and often a shortening of the total cycle; these mares may have a missed oestrus unless teasing is started before 17 days and may then be considered to have had a long interoestrus period. If oestrus is detected at the heat after infection, discharge may be absent as a result of the following sequence of events:

(i) infection which persists into the luteal phase, i.e. in this sort of mare, becomes more aggressive because circulating progesterone further reduces the resistance of the endometrium thus allowing enhanced bacterial multiplication.

(ii) bacterial endometritis appears to stimulate premature production of uterine prostaglandin.

(iii) this causes early regression of the CL (as soon as 7 days after ovulation).

(iv) the consequent reduction in progesterone removes the inhibition on the uterine defence process, and allows the cervix to relax so that pus can drain out.

NB, this condition is not easy to diagnose but should be suspected if:

the mare discharges during interoestrus

the mare returns to oestrus before 17 days or has short interovulatory period (i.e. less than 19 days)

the mare has palpable dilations in the uterus, a history of previous infection, or fluid in the uterine lumen when examined by ultrasound

the mare has muco-purulent discharge 7−8 days after parturition

13.3 Pyometra

This term is usually reserved for situations where chronically accumulated pus causes marked uterine distention; however, ultrasound examination can identify small pockets of pus which can confuse the definition.

• pyometra is not common in the mare because endometritis usually causes luteolysis with consequent relaxation of the cervix and drainage of the exudate

• the development of pyometra usually requires two lesions:

(i) endometritis.

(ii) cervical abnormality (fibrosis or adhesions) which prevents drainage; however, some cases of pyometra associated with a normal cervix have been described.

• diagnosis of pyometra is usually by rectal palpation of a large, thick walled, distended uterus; this can be difficult to differentiate from pregnancy without use of ultrasound

• the mare may have a slight intermittent vulval discharge (associated with times when the cervix is trying to relax, i.e. oestrus); this occurs when the cervix is slightly patent.

• oestrous cycles may be:

(i) short to normal in length; in this case luteolysis is usually being caused by premature prostaglandin release from the uterus.

(ii) long; this is rare and occurs in chronic cases where the uterus is so damaged that it can no longer release prostaglandin and therefore the CL persists.

• treatment is difficult but mainly relies on:

(i) induction of luteolysis — this may cause sufficient cervical relaxation to allow some drainage to occur.

(ii) trying to catheterize the stenosed cervix and drainage of the uterus, by suction or siphonage.

(iii) three or four daily treatments (drainage and antibiotics) may be necessary, between each of which the uterus will involute further. Antibiotic treatment of the uterus should be carried out for 5 days after complete drainage.

(iv) induce luteolysis as soon as possible after the next ovulation.

(v) attempts may be made to resolve cervical lesions, but most mares with pyometra have very poor breeding prospects and the condition often recurs if the mare is covered again.

13.4 Venereal bacteria (also see 16.2, 16.3)

• the organism of contagious equine metritis (CEMO), also called *Taylorella equigenitalis* (formerly *Haemophilus equigenitalis*) and some strains of *Klebsiella pneumoniae* and *Pseudomonas aeruginosa* are considered to be venereal

• when deposited in the uterus of normal mares they cause an active inflammation (i.e. in the absence of pneumovagina, reduced uterine resistance or cervical lesions)

• this endometritis is persistent and may last for more than one cycle before it eventually resolves

• this causes infertility because:

(i) luteolysis is premature, and the mare returns to heat repeatedly and usually early.

(ii) the mare is a source of infection to the stallion, who transmits the organisms to other mares.

(iii) handlers and veterinary surgeons may also act as disease transmitters to other mares.

• some mares, which may or may not have shown signs of previous endometritis, act as carriers of venereal disease

• they harbour the organisms in the vestibular area, particularly the clitoral fossa and sinuses

• although they show no signs of infection, they are potentially dangerous because:

(i) covering or gynaecological examination may carry the organisms forward into the uterus, causing endometritis.

(ii) the stallion may transmit these bacteria to other mares.

• it is interesting to note that:

(i) stallions may harbour the organisms all over the penis (including the urethral fossa) and in the distal urethra, but show no signs of disease.

(ii) CEM does not cause abortion, and mares have been known to discharge infected exudate from the vulva but have normal foals — the source of the discharge has not been ascertained.

(iii) both sexes of foals from mares harbouring CEM in the distal genital tract can acquire the organism in their own genital areas. The mode of transmission is unknown as the foal is born in the intact amnion and doesn't contact the mare's genital tract during normal parturition.

NB, CEM is now a notifiable disease.

14 / Swabbing techniques and diagnosis of endometritis

Swabbing of the mare's genital tract is carried out either to indentify unaffected carriers of venereal pathogens, i.e. clitoral swabs (and penile swabs in stallions) or to diagnose uterine infection by cytological and cultural techniques.

14.1 Clitoral swabbing (for venereal disease carriers)

• in thoroughbreds the regulations for clitoral swabbing are described in the code of practice for controlling CEM (Appendix 1)

• mares from which CEMO, *Klebsiella spp.* or *Pseudomonas spp.* are isolated should not be covered until they have been treated and reswabbed negative; however, only capsule types 1, 2 & 5 of Klebsiella and some strains of pseudomonas are pathogenic and the course of action taken depends on the policy of the stud

• before taking the swab the mare should be adequately restrained (**3.1**) and standing in a position where her vulval area is well illuminated

• ideally an assistant should hold the tail to one side; if more than one mare is to be swabbed, the assistant should wear a separate disposable glove/sleeve for each mare

• if faeces have caused gross contamination of the vulva wipe with a dry paper towel, do not otherwise cleanse the area

• the veterinary surgeon should also wear a sleeve on the hand used to evert the ventral vulva and expose the clitoris

• a small swab (Fig. 14.1) is used to swab both the clitoral fossa and the central clitoral sinus (Fig. 14.2); in high risk mares, as defined in the code of practice, two swabs should be used, one for each site.

• venereal pathogens live in smegma so that collection of this material from the sinus or fossa is advantageous

• clitoral swabs are immediately placed in Amies or Stuart's transport medium and sent to an approved laboratory to arrive during the working week

• if the swab is moistened, sterile water should be used and *not* saline

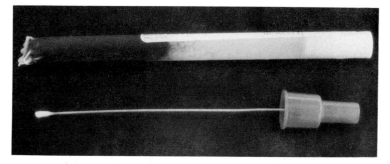

Fig. 14. 1. A swab (and tube of transport medium) suitable for penetrating the clitoral sinuses.

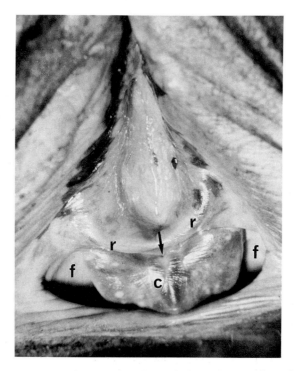

Fig. 14.2. Clitoral area of the mare: **c**, clitoris; **f**, clitoral fossa; **r**, clitoral frenulum; the arrow points to the opening of the central clitoral sinus.

• clitoral swabs are often not taken properly because:

 (i) the swabs may be taken before the mares goes to the stud, in order to save time at the stud, by practitioners who are not conversant with the technique.

 (ii) inadequate assistance makes proper swabbing very difficult, e.g. if no one is available to hold the tail.

 (iii) penetration of the clitoral sinus usually evokes a pain-stimulated response from the mare; poor restraint can therefore prevent proper swabbing.

 (iv) large swab tips may not penetrate the clitoral sinus.

 (v) failure to preserve the swab in correct transport medium and immediate dispatch to the laboratory necessitates reswabbing.

14.2 Uterine swabbing

• collection of material from the uterus is essential for the diagnosis of endometritis

• mares may be swabbed before covering to ensure that the uterus is not inflamed, and to check further for venereal pathogens

• the common organisms isolated from mares with non-specific endometritis are β-haemolytic streptococci (BHS) and *Escherichia coli*; over 90% of infections are caused by one or both of these organisms. Occasionally α-haemolytic streptococci, non-haemolytic streptococci, staphylococci and *Proteus vulgaris* are found in mixed infections with BHS and *E. coli*

• these organisms, along with many others, are normal inhabitants of the vulva and vestibular area, and only colonize the uterus for reasons previously described.

• an ideal swabbing technique should therefore ensure that:

 (i) the swab enters the uterus.

 (ii) the swab collects bacteria from nowhere other than the uterine lumen.

 (iii) the technique can be carried out with minimal assistance.

• intrauterine swabbing techniques are of two types, i.e. via a speculum or using a manual, guarded swab

• the former approach is most common in the UK and involves dilating the vagina and visualizing the cervix with a vaginal speculum

Speculum examination (13.6)

• ease of visualization of the cervix with a speculum depends on

the type of speculum used, the type of horse examined and the amount of assistance available
• speculae are of two basic types:

The metal speculum
The metal speculum, e.g. the duck-billed (Russian) speculum (Fig. 14.3a). This was commonly used until recently; the advantage of this speculum is that the anterior vagina can be fully dilated giving a good view of the cervix to allow passage of a swab into the cervical lumen. A disadvantage of this speculum is that it requires sterilization between mares; this can be achieved by having a number of speculae on the stud and sterilizing in boiling water; short-term chemical sterilization is inadequate.

Also a separate light source is necessary for illumination of the anterior vagina; if this is introduced into the vagina it is prone to contamination and should be protected.

Tubular speculae
Tubular speculae are of two types:
1   The most commonly used is the plastic tube which separately houses a protected light source (Fig. 14.3b, c). The tube sleeve can be resterilized although it eventually becomes opaque.
2   Recently a cheap disposable cardboard tube, slightly longer than the plastic version, has become available; a separate light source is necessary when using this method (e.g. a pen torch) — the tube is 'silvered' to aid illumination.
• both types have the advantage of allowing sterile examination of mares, but the view down the speculum is limited by the narrowness of the tube; occlusion by the passage of a swab down the tube limits vision. NB, All intrauterine swabbing techniques using a speculum are potentially inaccurate because:
• the cervix can become contaminated with bacteria carried forward from the vulval lips and vestibule on the speculum as thorough sterilization of the vestibule is impossible; the swab will collect these transferred organisms during examination
• contamination of the swab by inadvertant movement of the mare can occur when adequate assistance is not available, e.g. to hold the tail and to steady the mare
• light sources are often unreliable and may flick on and off
• it may be difficult to ensure that a swab has been passed through

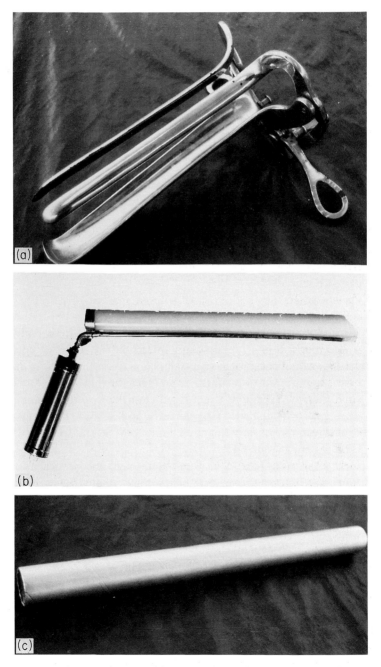

Fig. 14.3. Three types of vaginal speculum. (a) Metal (Polanski's) speculum. (b) Resterilizable plastic tube speculum with light source. (c) 'Silvered' disposal plastic tube.

the cervical canal and into the uterus; this is most easy during oestrus but even then the canal may be convoluted and although patent may prevent easy passage of a swab
• in particular the precision with which uterine swabs can be taken depends heavily on the quality and quantity of lay assistance available - the average practitioner may only have one or two (inexperienced) helpers for this procedure, in which case less than optimal standards are inevitable

Swabbing technique
• whatever type of speculum is used, the vulva should be thoroughly cleaned beforehand and the tail covered with a disposable bandage or sleeve
• some authorities advocate the use of clean water and cleansing material to remove gross contamination (this helps to prevent bacterial resistance to antiseptics), others advocate use of various antiseptic substances
• the speculum may be lubricated with an antiseptic-free gel (e.g. K−Y jelly) or warm water
• initially the speculum should be introduced through the vulval lips and pushed in a cranio-dorsal direction; after 5−10 cm a constriction (at the vestibulo-vaginal junction) is reached and further pressure is required to push the speculum past this
• thereafter the speculum is advanced cranially into the vagina
• during oestrus the body of the cervix is on the floor of the vagina and the external os is recognized as a spot or slit from which diverging oedematous folds radiate
• ideally the swab should be directed through the cervical canal without touching any other part of the tract, rotated a few times, and withdrawn in the same manner
• if the vagina remains collapsed after insertion of the speculum (i.e. air does not enter the vagina) visualization of the cervix is very difficult

Alternative technique
• the alternative method of swabbing is to use a guarded technique; this is not commonly used but has the advantage of being easy and accurate
• the swab is housed in a plastic, metal or cardboard tube (the guard); Figure 14.4 shows examples of these

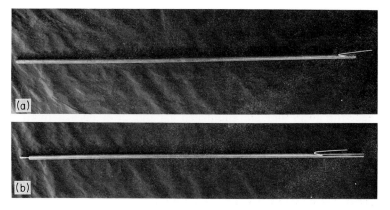

Fig. 14.4 One type of guarded intra-uterine swab. (a) Swab protected. (b) swab exposed.

• the operator uses a sterile sleeve, and places the guard tube (containing swab) along his/her dry, clean arm, inside the sleeve
• the knuckles of the hand (sleeve) are lubricated with sterile jelly and the arm is inserted into the vagina, the cervix is located and the index finger is inserted along the os
• the guard tube is advanced alongside this finger and finally pushed through the finger of the sleeve when further progression is impeded
• ideally the guard tube emerges from the sleeve at the tip of the index finger; in practice the point of penetration is usually within the cervical canal
• rupture of the sleeve should be sudden as very slow pressure stretches the sleeve excessively and may result in a thin film of plastic covering the end of the guard tube and subsequently masking the swab
• once the guard tube has entered the uterus and has advanced further than the tip of the index finger, the swab is expelled gently
• when resistance is met the swab is rotated several times and withdrawn into the tube; excess forward pressure results in endometrial damage as the swab will contact the uterus immediately after it leaves the guard tube
• the guard tube is now retracted into the sleeve and the arm withdrawn
• the advantages of this method are:
 (i) no assistance is required, e.g. to hold the tail.

(ii) the operator does not have to stand directly behind the mare.

(iii) contamination is minimal.

(iv) entry into the uterus is ensured.

• disadvantages are:

(i) the state of the cervix is not assessed visually.

(ii) bacteria may be introduced into the uterus; these do not contaminate the swab and are eliminated rapidly by a normal mare in oestrus. However, problem mares, and those swabbed in the luteal phase may have a subsequent endometritis.

• any intrauterine technique, therefore, should only be carried out during non-luteal phases; breach of the cervix in pregnant mares will almost invariably cause pregnancy failure.

14.3 Processing the swab

Uterine (endometrial) swabs may be used for:

Cytological examination

• if this is to be carried out it is best done by immediately rolling the swab gently onto a dry sterile slide, the swab can then be used for bacteriology

• the smear may then be air, heat or chemically fixed depending on facilities; swabs which are placed in transport medium and used later for smears may have lost cellular material. Alternatively two swabs may be taken (the second is used for cytology)

• various methods of staining are available — Leishman's, 'Diff Quik', methylene blue and gram's are simple and adequate; pre-stained slides are also useful (the main purpose of staining the smear is to show up polymorphonuclear leucocytes (PMN); trichrome stains are more complicated)

• the smear is examined for (Fig. 14.5)

(i) neutrophils (PMN); these are not present in the normal uterine lumen and indicate inflammation.

(ii) eosinophils are occasionally seen in endometritis.

(iii) endometrial epithelial cells indicate that the swab entered the uterus or contacted exudate from the uterus; squamous epithelial cells come from the cervix and vagina.

Bacteriological culture

• all swabs should be placed in Amies' or Stuart's transport medium unless they are to be plated out immediately; this is

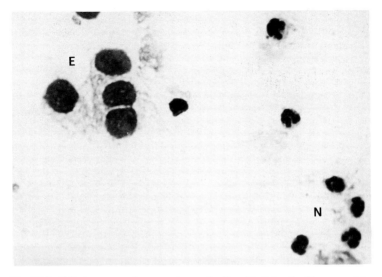

Fig. 14.5. Cells in a smear from uterine swab: E, epithelial cells; N, neutrophils.

essential when culture is for CEMO and desirable for all swabs; swabs which have dried in transit are useless (staphylococci, diphtheroids and fungi survive mild dessication)
• all swabs should be dispatched to the laboratory immediately; if this is by post the swabs ideally should not be taken just before the week-end
• clitoral swabs must always be placed in transport medium; if the swab needs moistening before use (also for penile swabs in stallions) sterile water and *not* saline should be used — dipping the swab in transport medium first is ideal.

14.4 Endometrial biopsy

Collection of the biopsy sample
• endometrial biopsies can be taken from mares at any time, except when complete fibrosis of the cervix is present; mid dioestrus is a good time as it minimizes misleading changes — avoid pregnancy!
• restrain the mare adequately (**3.1**), bandage the tail and cleanse and dry the vulva
• locate the cervix manually *per vaginam*, and dilate it with a finger; pass a sterile basket jawed forceps (Fig. 14.6) into the uterine lumen, and position so that the cutting jaw faces dorsally

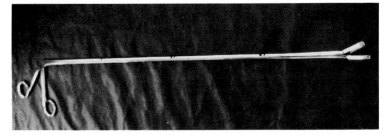

Fig. 14.6. Basket-jawed uterine biopsy instrument.

• a biopsy of the dorsal body can then be taken 'blind' by lifting the open jaws of the forceps, closing quickly and giving a 'tug', or the uterus can be located *per rectum* and the jaws of the instrument guided to the junction of body and horn
• considerable traction may be required to sever the biopsy, as the instrument does not cut cleanly
• contrary to initial fears:
  (i) it is virtually impossible to rupture the uterus.
  (ii) haemorrhage is rarely significant.
 (iii) the mare appears not to feel the procedure.

Processing the sample
• remove the tissue from the basket gently with a hypodermic needle
• immerse immediately in buffered formal saline or Bouin's fixative; the latter penetrates the tissue rapidly but the specimen should be removed in 24 hours
• sections may be stained with haematoxylin and eosin, or more specialized stains, e.g. van Giesen for fibrous tissue.

Interpreting the biopsy
• endometrial biopsies are more useful as a diagnostic rather than prognostic aid and accurate interpretation requires experience.
• physiological changes include:
  (i) oestrus — tall ciliated epithelial cells and active glands which may contain secretions, and may be separated by interstitial oedema.
  (ii) dioestrus — low cuboidal epithelium with small inactive glands.
 (iii) anoestrus — inactive epithelium and sparce glands; this may be mistaken for atrophy.

• pathological changes include:

(i) acute inflammation — neutrophil and occasionally eosinophil infiltration

(ii) chronic infiltrative inflammation (probably due to repeated bouts of acute inflammation) — mononuclear cells (histiocytes, lymphocytes and plasma cells) in the stroma

(iii) chronic degenerative change — layers of fibrous tissue (lamellae) round 'nests' or dilated glands and diffuse stromal fibrosis; may also get dilated lymphatic lacunae

(iv) atrophy, hypoplasia, hyperplasia, tumours etc. NB, mares with chronic endometrial change may still conceive.

15 / Treatment and prevention of endometritis

15.1 General considerations

• a normal transient endometritis occurs after covering and often after foaling; this is due to bacterial contamination, but post-covering endometritis may also be a reaction to seminal proteins

• it is considered that endometritis is usually caused by bacteria or yeasts and antibiotic therapy is therefore used

• however, methods of treatment are many and varied because the relative merits of intrauterine versus other routes of antibiotic treatment have not been extensively investigated (if i.m. or i.v. therapy is adopted, general recommendations for dose and length of treatment should be adopted)

• if intrauterine therapy is used, several aspects should be considered but there is no universally accepted method of treatment; the various criteria to be considered are:

(i) which antibiotic should be used; usually there is insufficient time for the results of a sensitivity test to be acted on. However, the most common pathogens are β-haemolytic streptococci, *E. coli*, staphylococci and anaerobes (*Bacteroides fragilis*); antibiotics of choice are therefore penicillin , streptomycin and possibly neomycin and nitrofurantoin (for anaerobes).

(ii) what volume of agent should be infused; traditionally the antibiotic is suspended in large (100–500 ml) volumes of water or saline on the assumption that this volume is optimal for filling the uterus; however, the chemical effect of such dilution on antibiotic efficacy is unknown, and present evidence suggests that most of the antibiotic introduced in this manner is expelled through the cervix soon after treatment. The author favours the use of 'neat' antibiotic on the assumption that the uterine lumen is only a potential space and therefore easily filled, and little of the agent is thereafter refluxed. Also, if the antibiotic is absorbed from the uterus it should theoretically return to this organ again in therapeutic concentrations in the blood for some time after treatment.

(iii) the length of intrauterine treatment is governed by the stage of the cycle.

(iv) what stage of the cycle is best for the treatment of endometritis?

• if a mare has no history of chronic endometritis, and is not suffering from pneumovagina, there is little theoretical reason why she should have a positive uterine culture in early oestrus; however, these mares do occur, and consideration should be given to the possibility that contamination of the swab has occurred (in this case cytological investigation is valuable)

• treatment may then be considered necessary at this stage, before the mare is covered, but since there is no evidence that endometritis is detrimental for sperm transport to the uterine tubes, the author is unsure of the necessity for withholding service.

15.2 Mares with impaired uterine resistance

The most common indication for treatment or prevention of endometritis is in the mare which cannot cope with infection introduced at covering. This may be dealt with by:

• using artificial insemination (**23.1**). Semen can be extended in a diluent containing antibiotic, and introduced into the uterus in an aseptic manner. This method is rarely used in the UK due to resistance by the Jockey Club and some breed societies

• minimal contamination technique; known susceptible mares have a large volume (100–500 ml) of semen extender, containing antibiotic, infused into the uterus immediately before service

• washing the mare's vulva and stallion's penis with water before coitus to remove gross contamination — the use of antiseptics is contra-indicated (**27.2**)

• antibacterial treatment after service; this is intended to allow the usual (if ineffective) inflammatory response to develop but to treat this so that the uterus is normal by the time the zygote enters it 5–6 days after ovulation:

(i) antibiotic may be instilled into the uterus for up to 3 days after ovulation; the uterus may be lavaged at this time with large volumes of normal saline to remove inflammatory exudate, with no detrimental effect on subsequent pregnancy.

(ii) treatment before ovulation may be wasted if a second covering becomes necessary.

(iii) augmentation of the uterine defence mechanism has been attempted using colostrum or plasma from mares. Until the cause of infection in these susceptible mares is known, the value of such therapy is speculative.

(iv) the use of indwelling uterine catheters can be beneficial where daily therapy is required, but these need suturing to the vulval area to reduce the likelihood of catheter loss, which nevertheless can occur; defecation on the catheter can cause ingress of infective material.

15.3 Chronic endometritis

This may be treated by:
• chemical cautery, e.g. 10% Lugols Iodine, although this may cause adhesions of the endometrium and damage to the opening of the uterine tubes
• physical cautery, i.e. scraping the endometrium with a special instrument
• intrauterine dimethyl sulphoxide.

15.4 Uro-vagina

Some mares, usually those that have pneumovagina (**13.2**), also pool urine in the cranial vagina — if urine gets into the uterus it may cause inflammation. Treatment is by:
• removing any vaginal urine before covering with a pipette, or giving the mare a fright to expel the urine due to increased abdominal pressure
• surgical reconstruction or lengthening of the urethral opening (Walker & Vaughan 1980).

15.5 Cystic endometritis

Glandular cysts are rarely large; lymphatic cysts are common in mares over 14 years of age, and may:
• cause no problems and go undetected
• be big enough to be mistaken for an early pregnancy, especially when at the base of a uterine horn; however, the absence of uterine tone would be suspicious (**8.3**)
• be mistaken for a pregnancy by ultrasound scanning, but they may not be the right size and shape or they may have been recognized previously; after 25 days an embryo should be seen in a pregnancy (**8.4**)

• numerous cysts may either prevent conception, or reduce the placental area sufficiently to effect the growth of the foal (**18.4**)
Treatment — cysts may be visualized using an endoscope (before covering) and ruptured using the biopsy facility of the instrument

15.6 Pyometra is rare (15.3)

• treatment consists of passage, if possible, of a catheter through the cervix and aspiration of pus (a vacuum pump is useful); this must be repeated daily, followed by antibiotic introduction
• after no more pus accumulates, antibiotic treatment is continued for 5 days. A total volume of 20 litres of pus is not unusual.

15.7 Post-partum metritis

Post-partum metritis is a very serious condition which occurs most often in mares with retained placenta and is particularly serious in heavy horses, when it should be regarded as an emergency (**22.9**).
• attempts to accelerate placental separation should be used (**23.1**)
• if placental separation is not complete (part of the non-pregnant horn is retained) or if post-partum metritis is suspected, at least daily lavage of the uterus is indicated; warm sterile saline (1−2 litres) should be introduced into the uterus, and immediately drained by siphonage; retention of some fetal membranes makes this difficult by blocking the drainage tube. A broad spectrum antibiotic should then be infused into the uterus — this should be effective against *E. coli* which is invariably present
• treatment is repeated until the pus and placental debris in the uterine exudate have disappeared
• supportive therapy with antihistamines and parenteral antibiotic is helpful
• despite all efforts some mares die due to toxaemia or irreversible laminitis and pedal-bone rotation

15.8 Pneumovagina

Treatment is surgical (**13.2**) but intrauterine therapy may be used before the operation to help the mare resolve her endometritis (she may also be immuno-incompetent).

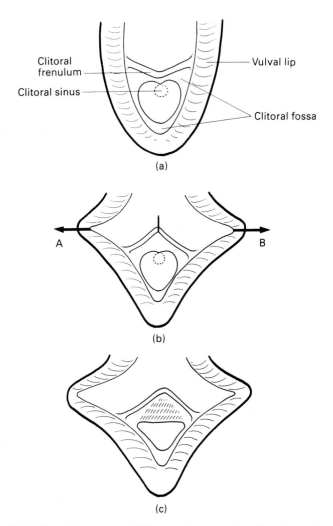

Fig. 15.1. Clitoral sinusectomy. (a) Restrain the mare, clean the vulva and note the anatomical sites. (b) Infiltrate the lateral vulval lips at A and B with local anaesthetic. These may then be retracted sideways using sutures, tissue forceps or retractors. Local anaesthetic infiltration into the clitoris and clitoral frenulum may not be necessary if the vulval block is adequate: retract the clitoral frenulum dorsally. (c) With rat-toothed forceps and curved scissors ablate the dorsal half of the clitoris, including the sinus; place this in transport medium for subsequent bacteriological investigation. Haemorrhage is usually minimal but may be staunched with an adrenalin swab.

15.9 Local clitoral treatment

After isolation of venereal pathogens (**13.4**) from the vulval and clitoral area these sites must be rendered free of these organisms before covering can begin.

- the area should be thoroughly washed with water containing an antiseptic (e.g. chlorhexidine) to remove smegma from the clitoral fossa and sinuses; these areas are then packed with any topical preparation (not containing cortico-steroid) of a suitable antibiotic — in the case of *Pseudomonas spp.* infection a 1 per cent silver nitrate aerosol may be used
- treatment is carried out daily for 5 days
- reswabbing after treatment is necessary (Appendix 1) to ensure complete removal of the potential pathogen.

15.10 Clitoral sinusectomy

Because of the inherent difficulties of swabbing and treating the clitoral area comprehensively, some mares in the past have remained positive for CEM without further covering.

- this led the authorities in North America to insist on removal of the dorsal part of the clitoris (including the sinuses) before mares could be imported
- the operation involves local analgesia of the area, either by direct infiltration into the body of the clitoris, or local block in the vulval labiae; desensitization of the clitoral frenulum is also necessary as this needs to be reflected dorsally to allow sight of the sinuses (Fig. 15.1)
- excision of the dorsal clitoris should be such as to remove the central and lateral sinuses (if present) completely and the tissue is submitted for laboratory examination and culture
- subsequent haemorrhage is usually minimal, but USA import regulations require follow-up local antibiotic treatment and swabbing, with supervision of the operation and post-operative treatment by an official from the Ministry of Agriculture.

16 / Viral causes of infertility

16.1 Viral abortion

Viral abortion is caused by an equine herpes virus (EHV1) and is also called rhinopneumonitis; it is not spread at coitus and aborted mares are soon free from the virus (the condition is discussed in 18.2).

16.2 Coital exanthema

• coital exanthema is also caused by a herpes virus (EHV3) and is transmitted venerally. Outbreaks are usually sporadic and the initial cause is often difficult to determine
• mares and stallions develop vesicular lesions on the vulva, vestibule and penis; these rupture and produce infected ulcers which usually heal well, although local antibiotic treatment may be prescribed to resolve secondary infection
• fertility is only affected if the mare or stallion is too 'sore' to achieve coitus; the condition usually resolves spontaneously in 14 days or so.

16.3 Viral arteritis

• viral arteritis is not at present in the UK
• it is a very severe disease which causes generalized malaise including fever, oedema and respiratory signs
• as a result of this, pregnant mares usually abort
• the virus may be spread venereally in stallion semen; these stallions remain persistent shedders of virus, but do not infect vaccinated mares.

17 / Problems during pregnancy

17.1 Definitions in pregnancy development (see also 7.1 − 7.3)

• pregnancy failure is a term used to denote failure of a fertilized egg to develop into a foal born live at term
• the consequences of such a failure depend largely on the stage of pregnancy at which death of the conceptus occurs
• various terms are used to describe the process of pregnancy development and pregnancy failure and its consequences; definitions of these terms are often not precise, but are best described as follows:

Embryo
This word is used to describe two entities:
• firstly after the fertilized egg (zygote) begins to divide, the resulting mass of cells is called an embryo
• at about 21 days after fertilization this mass of dividing cells has differentiated into those which are going to develop into the membranes and umbilical cord, and those which are going to form the new individual
• once this potential individual separates itself from the surrounding membranes, it is also called an embryo.

Fetus
• the embryonic tissue which is destined to become a foal grows slowly initially, because the elements within it are moving and rearranging themselves
• this primitive organization of organ precursors is called organogenesis and the developing individual is known as an embryo until the process is complete (in the horse about 40 days)
• thereafter the potential foal is called a fetus.

Conceptus
This is a blanket term and refers to all the products of conception throughout pregnancy, i.e. to the developing embryo or fetus plus its membranes and fluids etc.

17.2 Resorption

The impression given by this word is that an established pregnancy is dissolved or digested and disappears with no trace:
• in fact, death of the embryo or fetus before about 4 months is usually followed by dehydration of the conceptus, i.e. all the fetal fluid (which constitutes the bulk of the conceptus) is resorbed into the mare's circulation, and the solid tissue (embryo/fetus and membranes) is dried out and degenerated due to autolysis (release of cell enzymes)
• the mare may not return to heat for some time. The products of resorption will be expelled, usually unnoticed, on return to heat
• the stage of pregnancy at which fetal death is followed by immediate abortion, rather than resorption, is difficult to define as these events are rarely observed.

17.3 Mummification

• once a fetus has acquired a recognizable skeleton, i.e. after 4 months, continued presence of a dead fetus in the uterus results in the same dehydration process that is characteristic of resorption. However, in this case the bones will remain intact and the dehydrated fetus, a mummy, remains recognizable
• this situation only occurs in mares in which one of twins has died, because death of a single foal causes abortion, unless the fetus becomes lodged in the cervix.

17.4 Abortion

Abortion means the expulsion of uterine contents before term. However:
• the dehydrated remnants of early pregnancy failure are likely to be voided unobserved
• fetal death is followed by abortion once the placenta has become responsible for progesterone production (**7.4**)
• abortion may occur in mares at grass and not be recognized because mares usually show no after effects of abortion, and predators soon scavenge the abortus and membranes
• because pregnancy length is so unpredictable in the mare, the stage at which premature expulsion of a fetus changes to normal term parturition is difficult to define, and subsequent description of

events may depend on clinical assessment of the foal's ability to survive
• stillbirth usually refers to a dead foal produced after 320 days
NB, all aborted fetuses or foals born dead or dying should be sent for expert *post-mortem* examination, especially where other incontact mares are at risk.

17.5 Pseudopregnancy

This word is used to describe the reproductive phenomena which occur in the mare after pregnancy failure between 15 and 120 days of gestation.
• pseudopregnancy type I occurs when the embryo dies before day 36
• pseudopregnancy type II occurs when fetal death occurs after day 36, i.e. during PMSG (eCG) production (**7.4**)
• the clinical features of these conditions will be described later.

17.6 Pregnancy failure

• This subject is best considered by itemizing events in chronological order.

1–5 days
• undoubtedly some fertilized eggs fail to develop further and die in the uterine (Fallopian) tube
• as is the case for unfertilized eggs, these never reach the uterus
• the percentage of such failures is unknown
• the mare has normal oestrous cycle unless other events cause complications.

5–15 days
• fertilized eggs enter the uterus about 5 days after ovulation
• failure to develop further may be due to several causes, but those known are:
• endometritis not only produces an environment (inflammation) unlikely to support pregnancy development, but also initiates premature lysis of the CL (**13.1**)
• recent ultrasound studies have shown that many mares pregnant at 9 days are no longer in foal at 15 days; this suggests unawareness

of pregnancy and the CL regresses at the normal time or prematurely;
cyclic oestrous behaviour is obviously resumed.

15–36 days
• if the mare recognizes that she is pregnant at 15 days the CL
(corpus luteum verum) persists and the mare does not return to
heat
• clinically, all the features associated with pregnancy develop in
the tubular genitalia (**7.1, 7.2**)
• pregnancy failure results in resorption
• palpably (and on ultrasound scan) the pregnancy bulge disappears
due to dehydration, but:
• all the other features of early pregnancy (closed cervix, tonic
uterus, persistent CL, follicular growth) persist
• the CL, which is responsible for those features (but cannot be
palpated) may last for 3–4 months
• this is pseudopregnancy type I
• natural demise of the CL, or its premature lysis by exogenous
prostaglandin will cause rapid return to oestrus and expulsion of
remnants of pregnancy (can this be called an abortion?)
• the induced heat should be as fertile as any other.

37–140 days
• during this period PMSG (eCG) is normally produced
• eCG complicates the endocrinological environment so that pregnancy failure during this period results in:
• continued production of eCG until the endometrial cups die
naturally (there is no known method of accelerating their demise)
• the resulting syndrome is known as pseudopregnancy type II
• for as long as hCG is produced the mare will not get in foal again
• two patterns of reproductive behaviour have been described during
pseudopregnancy type II:
 (i) in ponies and some thoroughbreds recurrent periods of oestrus
occur with follicular development, but follicles become luteinized
(i.e. produce progesterone) without ovulating.
(ii) in some thoroughbreds the ovaries become small and quiescent
and the mare enters a period of anoestrus.

140 days to term
• the time when this period begins and the previous one ends is

very variable because of the individual differences in the length of time that hCG remains in the circulation (60–200 days)
- fetal death after hCG disappears from the blood is characterized by abortion because:
  (i) hormonal control of pregnancy at this stage is exercised by the fetus and placenta.
  (ii) fetal death is followed by a rapid drop in circulating oestrogen, and cessation of progesterone production.
  (iii) these changes cause cervical dilation and myometrial contractions which ensure expulsion of the fetus and usually also the membranes
- because of the ease of abortion, mares rarely show signs of malaise and often abort unnoticed
- after abortion the mare will come back into heat quite rapidly if this occurs in summer or spring, or may go into winter anoestrus if pregnancy fails in winter
- fertility after abortion should be good, but:
  (i) retained placenta may be more common than after normal birth.
  (ii) bacterial causes may leave residual infection which requires resolution before conception can occur.
  (iii) abortion of twins may delay subsequent conception, presumably because of overdistention of both uterine horns.

Premature and dysmature
Foals born before 320 days of gestation are arbitrarily defined as premature, although many of these survive; foals born after 320 days are sometimes weak and appear unprepared for extrauterine life — these are said to be dysmature.

18 / Causes of pregnancy failure

18.1 Bacterial infection

• the presence of bacteria in the uterus after fertilization prevents pregnancy development as previously described (**13.1**)
• it is unlikely that bacteria which enter the uterus at this early phase can persist and cause pregnancy failure later on
• in the latter half of pregnancy it is common for both bacteria, yeasts and other fungi to enter the uterus via the vagina
• the major cause of this is the mare developing pneumovagina due to loss of weight with subsequent vulval distortion (**13.2**)
• bacteria enter the vagina causing inflammation, which eventually spreads forward to the uterus
• the organisms which most commonly prevent early pregnancy establishment are β-haemolytic streptococci and coliforms
• these organisms and many others including aspergillus have been implicated in late abortion.
• entry of bacteria into the uterus causes:

Localized placentitis (placental inflammation)
• if transient does not spread or endanger the life of the fetus
• evidence of such an episode is seen at term when the allantochorion round the cervix is noticed to be devoid of villi and either thinned, or thickened with calcium deposits; there are histological signs of inflammation
• affected pregnancies may be long due to impaired placental function and reduced fetal nutrition

Extensive placentitis
• affects sufficient placental area seriously to retard development of the fetus, resulting in eventual abortion
• placental lesions are obvious and the aborted fetus may be small for gestation length

Bacteraemia or septicaemia
• entry of organisms into the uterus via the mare's blood stream, or more commonly via the cervix, can result in immediate transferral

to the fetus, with bacteraemia or septicaemia causing fetal death and abortion

18.2 Viral infection

• equine Herpes virus 1 (EHVI) or rhinopneumonitis virus causes abortion in mares (especially sub type 1)
• the virus also causes respiratory disease; this is most noticeable in horses (foals and yearlings) which meet the virus for the first time
• it may also cause paresis with ataxia, tail flaccidity and urine dribbling, or a fatal paralysis
• clinical signs of EHVI infection of the respiratory tract are not distinguishable from those caused by other viruses (and secondary bacterial infection), i.e. nasal discharge, transient pyrexia and physical depression
• animals which have previously met EHVI may become temporarily viraemic without showing clinical signs (usually older animals)
• source of virus is:
 (i) clinically affected animals; nasal secretions contain virus in animals which are both obviously infected and those which fail to show clinical signs.
 (ii) aborted fetus and their membranes.
 (iii) infected foals which are born live at term but which shed virus for the first week of life.
 (iv) mares which have aborted; these shed virus from the genital tract for only a short period, and can be covered after one month.
 (v) unsuspected virus shedders.
• the epidemiology of the disease is complicated by latency.
     after viraemia, virus can remain dormant (latent) in the reticuloendothelial cells of clinically normal animals for an unspecified length of time.
     activation of virus may be caused by stress or other factors.
     in pregnant mares this results in shedding and viraemia in the foal with subsequent abortion.

Diagnosis of EHVI infection
• there is no test to detect latent carriers
• viraemia is followed by a short lived rise in circulating complement fixing antibodies (70 days); serum neutralizing antibody remains elevated for longer

• virus isolation can be carried out on nasal secretions and fetal tissue
• post-mortem examination of aborted fetuses usually reveals fluid in the abdomen and thorax and necrotic foci in the liver; lesions are also found in the spleen, adrenal gland and thymus
• virus can be demonstrated in fetal lungs, liver and thymus by fluorescent antibody test on snap-frozen tissue
• these organs, particularly liver, contain intranuclear inclusion bodies

Epidemiology of EHVI
• foals and yearlings usually first contract the disease by contact with infected peers or adults suffering recrudescence after latency
• pregnant mares are usually infected by:
 (i) clinically infected youngsters.
 (ii) abortus of other mares.
 (iii) infected foals born at term may excrete virus for up to 9 days and may appear normal.
 (iv) clinically normal excreters.
• It is not known whether:
 (i) a mare can be carrying virus at time of conception, and abort later.
 (ii) aborted mares go into a further period of latency, but clinical experience suggest this is not so.
• mares which contract the virus during pregnancy will usually show no respiratory signs (due to anamnestic response); therefore the time at which aborting mares had contracted the virus is unknown, unless samples are available for serology
• abortions can occur as early as 7 days after exposure to virus and are usually seen after 5 months of gestation

Control of EHVI infection (Appendix 1)
Hygiene
• keep weaned foals and yearlings away from pregnant mares
• it is impractical on large studs to keep pregnant mares singly, but groups should be as small as possible and isolated from each other — this still may not prevent infection
• aborted fetuses and membranes should be sent for post-mortem examination where economically feasible
• all other products of abortion and contaminated bedding should be burned

- aborted mares should be isolated for at least 1 week with strict control of admission to the box and routine hygienic measures
- outside mares should not be allowed onto infected premises until at least 1 month after the last abortion
- similarly, resident animals should not be allowed to leave
- loose-boxes should be steam-cleaned and disinfected after being vacated by an aborting mare.

Vaccination
- two vaccines against EHVI are currently available in the UK, one dead and one attenuated
- only the dead vaccine is licenced for use in abortion protection
- experimental evidence casts doubt on their efficacy, but experience in the USA shows that regular and frequent vaccination reduces the incidence of abortion, and in particular prevents abortion storms
- vaccination should be considered where the cost relates favourably to the potential value of the foals at risk
- vaccination frequency is under review but should be as stated by the manufacturer
- ideally all horses on a premises should be vaccinated

18.3 Twinning (see also 7.7 and 20.1–20.3)

- basically, the mare's placenta is structurally simple, and requires occupation of the whole endometrial surface
- twin pregnancies pose a problem because two fetuses are trying to develop from a placental area designed for one (where the membranes of the two pregnancies meet, there is no placenta)
- in early pregnancy there appears to be a mechanism for causing death of the smaller of twins in some cases; this reduces the scale of later problems
- as pregnancy advances, the nutritional requirement of the fetus increases
- this demand is double in twin pregnancies, but one fetus usually receives a larger share to the detriment of the other
- the emaciated fetus eventually dies; presumably however, until this time it and its placenta have been contributing to the hormonal environment which sustains the pregnancy
- death of one fetus usually upsets hormone production sufficiently (basically progesterone production falls below a critical level) to allow cervical relaxation and myometrial contractions, i.e. abortion

- degeneration (autolysis) of the dead fetus is rapid at body temperature so that even a short interval between death of one fetus and abortion causes a marked change in the smaller fetus
- aborted twins have focal inflammatory foci in the liver which may indicate an immune mechanism in pregnancy failure.

18.4 Miscellaneous

- if the cause of an abortion is not investigated, it is easy to implicate some previous event, e.g. thunderstorm, kick by another horse, change in management, excess exercise, vaccination, worming etc.
- in most cases, in the author's opinion, these are merely incidental events, but being able to apportion blame is an understandable desire for the disappointed mare owner
- running the mare with a gelding does not cause abortion unless the gelding is 'riggy' and continually covers the mare (28.2)

Causes of abortion

Some causes of abortion are:

- twisting of the umbilical cord; when the cord is tightly wrapped around the trunk or a hind limb it is probable that the circulation may be impeded sufficiently to cause fetal death

(i) twisting the cord 'on itself' may be the result of fetal distress during an abortion, or may directly cause fetal death over a long period

(ii) evidence of previous (non-fatal) umbilical torsion is often seen when the urachus (thin walled) is dilated due to accumulation of urine or the bladder is grossly distended

- fetal abnormalities, e.g. hydrocephalus, occasionally stimulate abortion
- chronic endometrial change reducing functional placental area sufficiently to cause fatal malnutrition of the fetus
- development of excess fetal fluid is very rare and may either stimulate abortion or necessitate therapeutic termination of pregnancy
- iatrogenic abortion is rare; drugs which are known to upset pregnancies in other animals are unlikely to be used in sufficient quantities in mares in late pregnancy (e.g. oxytocin, prostaglandin, xylazine etc.)
- severe malnutrition at 20−30 days may cause resorption.

19 / Other abnormal events during pregnancy

19.1 Uterine torsion

• this can occur at any time during late pregnancy but is most common close to term
• the uterus twists about its long axis to between 90 and 360 degrees
• the mare shows typical signs of moderate to severe colic
• diagnosis is by examination *per rectum*; if the twist is anti-clockwise the right broad ligament can be felt stretched to the left over the dorsal surface of the uterus and vice versa
• the prognosis for the foal is poor because of interference to the blood supply to the uterus (due to compression of the major vessels)
• the prognosis for the mare depends on the speed of diagnosis and treatment
• treatment is correction of the torsion via laparotomy, usually under general anaesthesia. If this is carried out in late gestation the pregnant mare may abort, but some will foal normally at term
• reduction of the torsion close to term is best followed by Caesarean section via the same laparotomy.

19.2 Ventral hernia

• rupture of the prepubic tendon occurs mainly in Shire and heavy horses in late pregnancy
• this is characterized by massive ventral swelling and oedema
• prognosis is poor although live foals may be produced by assisted delivery after parturition induction (**19.7**) or Caesarean section (**24.5**).

19.3 Pseudopregnancy (17.5)

• early embryonic and fetal deaths result in physiological events which usually mimic continued pregnancy, i.e. pseudopregnancy
• however, by the end of the fifth month after conception, the pseudopregnant mare becomes capable of having normal oestrus cycles

• some mares, thought to be pregnant, put on weight and appear to have maintained gestation until examination at, or after, expected term shows they are non-pregnant

• weight increase in this case is due to over feeding (because of expected pregnancy); there is no physiological basis for 'pseudo-pregnancy' as there is in the bitch in late gestation

• mares (and fillies) may 'bag up' and even lactate at any time during their reproductive lives; this may be associated with increased feeding, especially grass, or other unknown factors

• lactation in non-pregnant mares usually stops without treatment, but may be curtailed by testosterone administration.

20 / Reducing infertility caused by twin pregnancy

20.1 Prevention of twin conception

1 Avoid covering mares with two follicles (may shorten next dioestrus with prostaglandin)

BUT

• mare may not be examined regularly enough for detection of two follicles
• mare may produce two follicles again at next heat
• may be too late in breeding season to avoid covering
• detection of two follicles may be impossible because:

(i) two follicles close to each other may feel like one large follicle on palpation, but can be recognized by scanning.

(ii) a follicle deep in the ovary may not be detected by palpation but would be seen by scanning.

(iii) a second follicle, unsuspected by palpation or scanning, may develop and ovulate rapidly during early dioestrus; if the mare was covered close to the first ovulation by a stallion with good fertility a second conception could occur.

2 Try to cover between two anticipated ovulations, on the assumption that the ovum released before covering is unlikely to be fertilized.

BUT

• covering after one of two ovulations can still result in twin conception
• both ovulations may occur between successive examinations
• such timing requires regular repeated examinations.

20.2 Diagnosis of twins

Manual palpation

• even under ideal conditions this can be no more than 66% accurate, as in about one-third of twin pregnancies both conceptuses are in the same uterine horn
• when twin pregnancies are in the same horn, they produce a single swelling at its base; contrary to expectations, this swelling feels no bigger than a single pregnancy of the same age

• twins which are located in separate horns (bicornual) are easier to detect as two distinct swellings

BUT

• pregnancy examination at 21 days may miss bicornual twins as the younger conceptus may not yet produce a palpable swelling
• bicornual twins may be more difficult to detect in the post-partum uterus, although this arrangement is less common than in barren or maiden mares
• the latest time for identification of bicornual twins by palpation is about 60 days — after this the two swellings become confluent; however, if twin pregnancy is to be terminated to give the mare a second chance to conceive during the current breeding season, diagnosis should be before day 33.

Ultrasound examination
• ultrasound gives a much more accurate diagnosis of twins than palpation, as the contents of the uterus are visualized, but it is *not* 100%
• scanning for twins usually results in a reduced insurance premium on the life of the unborn foal
• twin pregnancies may be identified as early as 14–16 days (high frequency transducers are most accurate at this early stage)
• wrong diagnosis may be caused by:
 (i) incomplete scanning of the uterus, which allows a twin to be missed.
 (ii) failure to recognize twins in the same horn because the plane of the ultrasound beam doesn't highlight the inter-conceptual wall; this can happen to the most experienced examiner, but is more common before both embryos become visible, i.e. about day 25.
(iii) cysts — these can easily be confused with pre-21 day pregnancies; regular repeated scanning is the only way to make the distinction accurately.
NB, after 60 days twin pregnancies are not diagnosable by palpation, and become rapidly more difficult by scanning.

20.3 Dealing with twin conception

• many twin conceptions result in the birth of a single healthy foal, i.e. 'nature' ensures that one pregnancy fails early enough to prevent interference with development of the other

• it has been postulated that this (resorption of one pregnancy) is much more likely after synchronized ovulations, compared with those that occur some time apart.

Coping with the problem

The clinician's dilemma is to decide whether and when to intervene — the decision must be made before day 33 if the mare is to stand a chance of getting in foal again during the same breeding season. Interference with a twin pregnancy can be by:

• abolition of the whole pregnancy by lysing the corpora lutea with prostaglandin — if initiated before day 36 the mare will usually have a normal subsequent heat with average fertility; attempts to do this after day 36 may not succeed and are unlikely to be followed by a fertile heat (**17.5**)

• manual rupture of one conceptus

(i) the smaller conceptus should always be chosen.

(ii) early conceptuses (16–20 days) are difficult to crush as they are mobile in the uterine lumen and cannot be fixed.

(iii) as the conceptus develops from day 21 greater pressure is required to rupture it and after day 25, repeated attempts may be required.

(iv) as pregnancy proceeds after day 21, manual disruption of one pregnancy is more likely to be followed by death of the other, i.e. complete pregnancy failure — this is attributed to prostaglandin release following uterine trauma, although other factors may be involved.

(v) bicornual pregnancies are most easily treated by this method, although gentle squeezing of two conceptions at the same site may be attempted in the hope that only one conceptus will be destroyed.

Assessing results

• successful twin management usually requires repeated examinations

• manual examinations after diagnosis and treatment can confirm or otherwise the continuance of pregnancy

• ultrasound examination is superior, in the hands of an experienced clinician, as the course of development of twins or a surviving singleton can be monitored more accurately.

21 / Retained placenta

21.1 Normal expulsion

• the physical contact between the allantochorion and the endometrium is relatively weak, so that placental separation occurs
rapidly after expulsion of the foal
• passage of the fetal membranes (cleansings, after-birth) is usually
complete by 3 hours post-partum
• however, it is traditional to consider that a problem exists if the
mare has not cleansed by 6 hours after birth — all these definitions
are arbitary
• after a normal birth the membranes which are hanging from the
vulva are the amnion (inner membrane) in which the foal was born,
and the enclosed umbilical cord; the amnion may contain pockets
of fluid (**7.3**)
• the weight of the amnion and cord result in the allantochorion
separating from the endometrium at the point where the cord is
attached to the allantochorion, i.e. at the base of the horn in which
the conceptus first developed
• progressive traction by the amnion causes complete separation of
the allantochorion, which becomes everted during the process (Fig.
9.1) and is passed inside-out.

21.2 Examination of the membranes

• always check that the expelled membranes are complete
• the amnion is usually torn but cannot be retained *per se*
• it is a white membrane containing large white blood vessels
• sometimes the amnion (and intra-amniotic umbilical cord) feels
rough due to small plaques of epithelial cells which appear to
contain glycogen; the significance of these is unknown but they are
considered to be normal
• the umbilical cord is usually twisted but not discoloured
• the allantoic portion of the cord contains four thick walled vessels
(two arteries and two veins)
• at the level of the attachment of the amnion, the two veins join
so that only three vessels traverse the amniotic cavity to the umbilicus

- abnormal twisting of the cord on itself (18.4) or round a fetal limb etc. may cause distortion or haemorrhage into surrounding tissue
- sacculations are sometimes seen in the amniotic cord — these are dilations in the urachus and probably reflect short periods of mild twisting
- the allantochorion should be spread out to ensure that all is present; its shape conforms exactly to that of the recently vacated uterus, i.e. a body and two horns
- the outer surface is matt due to villi and is red; differing intensities of colour occur normally due to hypostatic congestion with blood which was not expelled through the cord
- the tips of the horns are avillous over a small (¼ cm diameter) area where the chorion was against the uterine openings of the fallopian tubes
- the tips of the horns (especially the larger one) may be smooth and thickened due to oedema; the cause is unknown but this is thought to be normal
- a haphazard arrangement of avillous areas, roughly forming a circle around the attachment of the umbilical cord, marks the position in the uterus of the now disappeared endometrial cups; there is also a small avillous area which coincides with the base of the cord — this marks the embryonic yolk-sac (bilaminar omphalapleur) placenta
- the internal (non-placental) surface of the allantochorion is shiny and contains a mass of recognizable blood vessels
- in a circular area round the attachment of the cord, and corresponding to the avillous area described previously, are little sacs on thin stalks (the chorio-allantoic pouches); these contain dead endometrial cup tissue and are normal
- the portion of the allantochorion almost invariably left behind is the tip of the smaller (non-pregnant) horn, followed by the tip of the pregnant horn
- often the horns (and less commonly body) are ripped and it may be difficult to decide whether membrane has been left inside or not.

21.3 Abnormal expulsion

- immediately after the mare has foaled, the amnion is hanging from the vulva to the level of the hocks or below

• this may cause the mare to kick back, thus endangering the foal, or may be trodden on causing abnormal tension with a result that the membranes may tear, or the uterus may prolapse

• to prevent this the membranes should be tied without exciting the mare, to a position above the hocks

• baler twine is ideal for this, although the procedure is difficult due to the very slippery nature of the membranes

• *never* cut the amnion and cord off, as they provide the normal traction to produce natural separation of the allantochorion — also the amnion will retract back into the vagina taking bacteria and dirt with it

• *never* attach weights to the amnion and cord or pull on them; excess traction may cause rupture of the membranes or uterine prolapse (**22.7**)

• retention of the membranes for more than six hours is often considered pathological because this sometimes results in metritis and laminitis, with fatal results

• these severe sequelae are most often seen in heavy horses, but are rarer in the lighter breeds (including thoroughbreds)

• however, because the literature is explicit as to these possibilities (because most of it was first written at a time when heavy working horses comprised the major part of the equine population), it is prudent to treat the condition as potentially serious

• most mares suffer little after effects in the presence of prolonged retention, whereas some heavy mares succumb to fatal sequelae even after prompt and thorough treatment

• all mares with retained placenta should be visited

• ensure that the mare is adequately restrained in full view of the foal, which should be protected should the mare move violently around the box

• bandage the tail and cleanse the vulva as best as possible (the emergent membranes make this difficult). Well washed arms are preferable to gloves as differentiation between the tissues involved may be difficult

• at this stage some part of the separating allantochorion may be visible at the vulva or palpable in the vagina

• when removing fetal membranes manually, the reinforcement of the physiological method, i.e. tension via the umbilicus, cannot be exploited as traction may cause ripping of the membranes

• if pieces of membrane are left in the uterus they are usually

impossible to reach due to the disproportionate size of the recently evacuated uterus compared to the clinician's arm
• separation of the allantochorion from the endometrium is therefore attempted from the cervical end of its attachment (Fig. 21.1)
• the torn (cervical) end of the CAM is grasped (this contains the umbilical cord and maybe some amnion) and gently pulled posteriorly
• usually there is enough 'give' for this then to be held by a second hand at the vulva
• at this stage the held allantochorion is twisted; this ensures that the force transmitted through the membranes is equally distributed throughout its attachment, i.e. that pieces of membrane are not pulled off piecemeal
• with the allantochorion under tension, the hand in the tract is inserted between the CAM and endometrium and moved in a circular manner to separate the two
• if separation is easy, i.e. the two components part like 'velcro' and there is no haemorrhage, then continued traction and tension on the exposed CAM will bring the more anterior portions of the uterus into reach for similar treatment

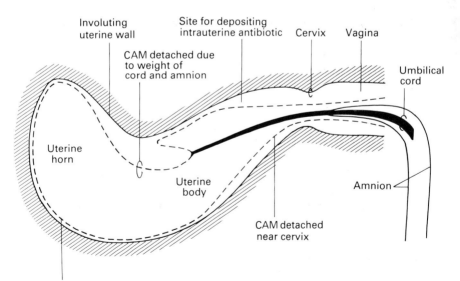

Fig. 21.1. Arrangement of the fetal membranes immediately after delivery of the foal (CAM; chorio-allantoic membrane).

- manual removal must be carried out with patience; the extent of success is difficult to determine — often the complete placenta separates and flops to the floor when least expected
- *however*, if manual removal is difficult, takes more than 10 minutes or causes haemorrhage, other treatments should be considered
- firstly, antibiotic may be infused into the uterus (see later), antihistamines given parenterally, and the mare revisited in 6–12 hours; several subsequent visits may be necessary before removal is complete
- secondly, oxytocin may be administered; some clinicians prefer this treatment as an initial approach
- ideally, an intravenous drip is established and 10–20 iu oxytocin given in 1 litre of saline over a period of one hour
- the uterine contractions thus stimulated will hasten placental separation and may result in less micro-villous necrotic material being left *in utero*
- this may be difficult if the mare is restless and is trying to 'nuzzle her foal'
- single doses of oxytocin (up to 40 iu) may be given i.m. but these are less physiological and large doses may cause excessive straining and uterine prolapse
- after a complicated cleansing, heavy mares should receive continued antibiotic and antihistamine treatment and daily uterine lavage
- this consists of infusing 500 ml warm sterile saline, and siphoning out the dark detritis
- similar treatment should be considered for mares which have retained some of the fetal membranes
- treatments should continue until the siphoned material is clear — if the aspirated material becomes purulent the mare has developed endometritis
- in the author's opinion, neat antibiotic at the parenteral dose should be inserted after any intrauterine post-partum interference
- if the membranes have not been expelled the location of the antibiotic should be chosen carefully, i.e. it must be deposited between the CAM and the endometrium
- this is because absorption through the now dead allantochorion is probably poor, and because the bacteria introduced by the examiner's arm are likely to be between the endometrium and the CAM (see Fig. 21.1)

- mares which have been slow to cleanse are less likely to conceive at the foal heat; if covering at this heat is seriously considered the mare should be examined *per rectum* and *per vaginam* before hand to assess involution (**10.3**).

22 / Other post-partum problems

22.1 Vulval and perineal trauma

• bruising of the vagina, vestibule and vulva commonly occurs during parturition
• deeper damage is only recognized if the mare is examined *per vaginam*; swelling of the vulval lips is often observed and usually resolves within a few days of parturition
• vulval and perineal tears may occur in any direction but usually result from:
(i) ripping at any angle either spontaneously or as a result of previous vulval closure which has not been opened.
(ii) tearing of a normal vulva due to a large foal.
• suturing is usually necessary, and can be carried out without local anaesthetic if the mare has foaled within the previous few hours.

22.2 Recto-vaginal fistula (24.3)

Occasionally the foal's foot penetrates the caudal rectum and causes severance of the vaginal roof and the rectal floor.
Thereafter relaxation of expulsive efforts may result in realignment of the fetal limb and subsequent normal birth:
• in this case the recto-vaginal lesion often heals to form a fistula which allows constant access of faecal material to the vagina
• this causes endometritis and can only be diagnosed by careful examination *per vaginam*
• treatment is difficult but relies on careful disection of the fistula *per vaginam* and repair of the vaginal roof by suturing — treatment may be as for perineal laceration.

22.3 Perineal laceration

Rupture of the rectum may be followed by continued straining and trauma, resulting in recto-vaginal severance to the perineum:
• post-partum, a rip between anus and vulva is evident, with gross contamination of the vagina/vestibule with faeces

• immediate treatment is antibiosis and supportive medication if necessary
• surgical treatment is delayed until the wound has healed by second intention, and the extent of the operative problem can be assessed
• under general anaesthesia (or local epidural block) an attempt is made to repair the vaginal roof, thus providing a reconstructed rectal floor
• several attempts may be necessary before an adequate surgical repair is achieved (Walker & Vaughan 1980)
• covering should be with-held until the next breeding season
• the anus may never function properly

22.4 Ruptures of the cervix and vagina *per se*

• these are rare and may result in peritonitis or pelvic abscess, depending on the site
• cervical damage is serious because subsequent fibrosis or adhesions (**13.3**) may compromise function and predispose to pyometra
• surgical treatment of cervical lesions is difficult and the prognosis for future fertility is poor

22.5 Uterine rupture

• this occurs occasionally due to continued contractions during either an apparently normal parturition or during dystocia
• if the mare's abdominal viscera are eventrated, diagnosis is easy
• uterine rupture may result in rapid onset of peritonitis and death despite supportive treatment (antibiotics, fluids etc.)
• occasionally the sequence of uterine involution and membrane expulsion may be such that peritoneal contamination does not occur, but adhesions between the uterus and adjacent viscera may form
• if initial diagnosis is easy, and surgical facilities are available, uterine repair may be successful via laparotomy

22.6 Haematoma

Rupture of the uterine vessels or their branches is not uncommon.
• smaller vessels bleed into the space between the myometrium

and its serosal covering until the build up of pressure produces haemostasis:

(i) in this case the mare may exhibit mild signs of colic after delivery.

(ii) examination sometime later will reveal a fluctuant or hard mass on the surface of the uterus.

(iii) resolution of the haematoma occurs slowly, and usually does not affect the ability of the mare to conceive again.

• extensive haemorrhage ruptures the uterine serosa

• the mare shows moderate to severe signs of colic with progressive anaemia

• diagnosis is difficult (the immediate post-partum uterus cannot be palpated in its entirety) and the outcome is usually fatal.

22.7 Uterine prolapse

• this is uncommon in the mare and may occur immediately after expulsion or due to traction on fetal membranes or straining

• the everted endometrium is very vascular and easily recognized as such

• fatal haemorrhage may occur if the uterus is traumatized

• epidural anaesthesia may be used but this often takes a long time to work and is usually unnecessary with adequate restraint of the mare

• the membranes should be removed and the uterus washed

• lifting the uterus helps to reduce congestion and facilitates replacement if help is available

• the uterus is 'fed back' from the vulval attachment (vagina) using a clenched fist and copious lubrication

• replacement is usually easier than in the cow and should be followed by insertion of a clean bottle or large volumes of saline to ensure complete eversion of the horns (saline should subsequently be siphoned off)

• suturing of the vulva is unnecessary, but may be requested

• supportive treatment involves antibiosis, antihistamines and maybe corticosteroids and calcium; oxytocin is contra-indicated as this stimulates further uterine contractions

• in heavy horses, daily uterine lavage and antibiosis is indicated (**21.3**)

• fatal toxaemia may occur despite treatment

22.8 Hypocalcaemia

• this is rare in the mare and usually occurs immediately pre- or post-partum
• the condition is more related to stress than calcium metabolism *per se*, and characteristically occurs in feral horses which have been housed prior to foaling
• severe signs are recumbancy accompanied by tetanic spasms
• mild cases involve slight hyperaesthesia and very dry faeces
• treatment is the slow infusion of calcium borogluconate to effect with continuous monitoring of cardiac activity.

22.9 Post-partum endometritis

• this condition is dealt with in Chapter 15.

22.10 Management of the engorged udder

• either at planned or unanticipated weaning, the best advice is inactivity
• restricting water and feeding hay only may reduce lactation
• milking and lavage of the udder only provide further stimulus for milk production and may initiate mastitis
• the mare may be uncomfortable for 24–48 hours post-weaning, but non-interference with the udder is advisable
• when mastitis does develop, stripping of the quarter (every 2–4 hours) is initially beneficial, with antibiosis
• when the udder is no longer hot (despite the degree of induration), milking should stop; usually the lack of attention to the opposite gland has reduced the rate of milk production.

23 / Manipulation of reproduction

23.1 Artificial Insemination (AI)

• the use of AI is limited in the UK because the authorities will not allow registration of thoroughbred foals born as a result of AI
• this is presumably because of the possibility of individual stallions being used to producing excessive numbers of foals, and because the system could be abused, with parentage subsequently being attributed to the wrong stallion; this latter objection is now eliminated by blood testing.

Advantages of AI
These are:
• insemination is easy in the mare; the insemination catheters can be passed into the uterus by manual guidance *per vaginam*, and if necessary the catheter can be directed *per rectum* to the tip of the uterine horn ipsilateral to the ovulating ovary
• one ejaculate can be split into several portions, especially if accurate insemination is carried out as just described
• busy stallions need only to be collected from once every two days under normal circumstances
• more mares can be inseminated from a particular stallion than by normal service
• semen can be transported more easily than the stallion, for mares some distance away
• semen can be stored for use after the death of a stallion
• dilution of semen in extender containing antibiotic reduces the risk of veneral (and other) disease (**13.4**)
• similar treatment to semen reduces uterine contamination for mares with poor uterine immunity (**13.2**)
• regular collection of semen from stallions allows constant checking of seminal quality and bacterial content.

Disadvantages of AI
These are:
• collection may be difficult or hazardous, especially if the stallion is not used to the procedure

• a mare in season is necessary, preferably one that stands quietly, although stallions can be trained to jump dummies and some can be collected from without mounting

• theoretically a stallion could become overused in a particular mare population

• wilful deceit could result in a mare being inseminated with the wrong, or erroneously labelled semen; however in the author's opinion this is no more likely or undetectable than covering a mare with the wrong stallion

• since collection and insemination is usually carried out by a veterinary surgeon, the cost would usually be increased.

Collection of semen

Semen is collected by:

1 An *artificial vagina* (*AV*). These are costly but provide an environment similar to the normal vagina (**26.3**).

• the stallion is allowed to mount a mare in heat, and his penis is directed into the AV

• most stallions accept the AV but some are very reluctant to ejaculate into it

• the collector is well-advised to wear protective foot and headwear

NB, this is the method of choice

2 *Rubber condoms or breeder's bags*. These are available in the USA, and are placed over the stallion's penis before he covers the mare; the condom is removed at dismount.

Plastic 'rectal' sleeves are sometimes placed over stallion's penis in a similar manner.

3 *Dismount sample*. This is the fluid ejaculated by many stallions during withdrawal, especially if the penis is still erect.

• if the stallion's penis goes flaccid whilst still in the mare's vagina, fluid often escapes from the vulva on withdrawal

• in either case it is composed mainly of viscous, seminal vesicle secretion

• if, however, adequate sperms are present for insemination of this material into a mare to be worthwhile, the advantages of disease control are negated

• evaluation of such a sample only gives a rough guide to its quality (**26.4**).

Treatment of stallion semen before AI
• if mares are close the raw semen can be inseminated within a short period of time if rapid cooling of the sample (causing 'cold-shock') is avoided; this does not reduce bacterial numbers in semen
• immediate dilution in an extender at 37°C should be made for problem mares, or where some delay in insemination is anticipated
• many extenders have been used for stallion semen, but one which is suitable and easy to make is: non-fat dried milk, 2.4 g; glucose, 4.9 g; crystalline penicillin 0.09 g; crystalline streptomycin, 0.15 g; sterile distilled water, 100 ml. 1 vol. semen: 3 vols extender
• if extended semen is slowly cooled to +4°C, viability should remain reasonable for 12−48 hours as long as the quality of the initial sample was good
• Deep-freezing of stallion semen can be carried out with post-thawing samples giving acceptable pregnancy rates. At present there are few indications for the use of this technique in the UK.

23.2 Embryo transfer

Non-surgical embryo transfer is possible in the horse.
• the technique of embryo collection is relatively simple, i.e. the embryo is flushed out of the mare's uterus 7 or 8 days after ovulation:
  (i) this requires the infusion and subsequent collection of physio-logical solution, which is introduced through the cervix of the conscious mare.
  (ii) the embryo is quite easily identified and can be inseminated into the uterus of a mare at the same stage of the cycle, using a specially designed pipette which ensures delivery of the embryo.
  (iii) scrupulous asepsis is essential during ovum insertion to avoid bacterial inflammation-induced luteolysis.
• the advantages of embryo transfer are:
  (i) embryos may be collected from a valuable mare which is thought to be otherwise unable to maintain a normal pregnancy, e.g. due to age, uterine damage, prepubic tendon rupture etc.
  (ii) several embryos may be collected from one mare of an endan-gered breed during one breeding season, thus increasing the number of foals of that breed born the following year.
  (iii) the technique helps with the understanding of fundamental physiological aspects of equine reproduction, e.g. when donkey embryos are transferred to horse mares etc.

• problems with embryo transfer in the mare are:

(i) superovulation is difficult to stimulate so usually there is only one embryo after each successful collection; research in this field may be fruitful in the near future.

(ii) due to the long follicular phase of the mare's oestrus cycle, it is very difficult to synchronize ovulations (i.e. between donor and recipient); it is therefore usually necessary to have several potential recipient mares for each donor.

(iii) this makes embryo transfer expensive because of the number of mares which must be kept and monitored closely for each possible success.

23.3 Micromanipulation of embryos

• the use of genetic engineering has had little impact on horse reproduction at present

• however, successful spliting of the mare egg, fertilized *in vitro*, with subsequent production of identical twins in two recipient mares has been reported

• further development in this field is likely.

24 / Dystocia

24.1 Definitions

Dystocia
Any problem which interferes with the normal birth of the foal.

Presentation
The direction the foal is facing relative to the long axis of the mare; this can be:
• anterior longitudinal, i.e. normal — the foal's head is presented towards the mare's vulva (preceded by the feet); a late pregnancy examination may often confirm this presentation
• posterior longitudinal, i.e. the foal is 'back-to-front' and the rump is presented first
• transverse — this implies that the foal lies at right angles to the mare's spine, i.e. it occupies both uterine horns. In reality the foal cannot lie transversely across the mare's abdomen and appears to be in a longitudinal presentation. Thus the uterus is distorted to accommodate this rare presentation.

Position
This describes the relationship between the foal's back and the mare's spine; normal birth is accomplished in the dorsal position, i.e. foal's back uppermost.
• during later pregnancy the foal may lie on its side (lateral position) or back (ventral position) but rotates during late first and early second stage labour — this may fail to occur during induced parturition.

Posture
The disposition of the neck and limbs, relative to the body.
• essentially these are either extended (as the neck and fore-limbs are in normal birth) or flexed
• hip-flexion in posterior presentation results in 'breach birth'
• flexion of the fore-limbs may be unilateral or bilateral and involve any joint, and may occur in normal limbs or those with tendon contractions

• head and neck flexion only occur in anterior presentation and may be associated with ankylosis (fusion) of the cervical vertebrae (wry-neck)
• unilateral or bilateral flexion of the hind limbs, when the foal is in anterior presentation results in the undiagnosable 'dog-sitting' position.

24.2 Significance of dystocia

• despite the long limbs of foals, dystocia is rare in the mare
• luckily, the most severe forms of malpresentation are the rarest
• sadly, dystocia usually results in death of the foal and maybe the mare because:
(i) the mare usually continues with expulsive efforts, even if the foal is 'stuck'
(ii) the placenta separates rapidly during labour and unless the foal can breath it soon loses its oxygen supply and dies
(iii) continued unproductive straining by the mare may cause damage to her reproductive tract
(iv) uterine damage during dystocia can cause fatal peritonitis or haemorrhage
(v) retained placenta, as a result of uterine inertia following dystocia can be fatal
(vi) uterine prolapse may occur

24.3 Recognition of dystocia

1   The foal is normally born in anterior presentation, dorsal position and extended (head, neck and forelimbs) posture.
2   Failure to observe the fluid filled amnion (which may be visible only during contractions) at the vulva after 5 minutes of second stage labour indicates that vaginal examination is necessary and may reveal:
• two feet (one anterior to the other) and a nose, i.e. normal birth — delay could be due to:
(i) feto-maternal disproportion or fetal oversize; this is rare in mares except the smaller breeds of pony
(ii) hydrocephalus impeding passage of the enlarged head through the cervix. This is rare.
(iii) slow relaxation of the cervix (after induction of parturition).

(iv) ineffectual straining. This is rare.

(v) dorsal deviation of one or both feet — if unrecognized and corrected this can cause recto-vaginal trauma (**22.2**, **22.3**).

(vi) slowness of the fetus to rotate into normal dorsal position — this is recognized by inability of the fetlocks to flex ventrally, but they will do so dorsally or laterally, and the limbs may be crossed.

• one foot and nose — carpal and/or shoulder flexion of one fore limb

• nose only — carpal and/or shoulder flexion of both fore limbs

• two limbs only; this could be:

(i) head and neck flexion — carpi flex in a ventral direction unless position is also wrong.

(ii) posterior presentation with hind-limbs extended; these flex in a dorsal direction and the hocks should be palpable — recognition of the tail will help diagnosis.

• nothing palpable in the vagina — this is serious and indicates:

(i) transverse presentation — may recognize fetal abdomen in the uterus.

(ii) posterior presentation with bilateral hip flexion (breech).

(iii) anterior presentation with bilateral limb and head/neck flexion.

• tough allantochorion identified — no fluid loss seen and vagina still relatively dry. Foal being born in CAM and placenta separating. NB, this must be distinguished from an unopened cervix; often an owner will misinterpret discomfort and grunting for second stage labour.

• very rarely, prolapse of the mare's bladder causes dystocia.

24.4 Non-surgical treatment of dystocia

Restraint

• Most mares are too concerned with foaling to worry about manipulation *per vaginam*

• however, due to discomfort the mare is disinclined to stand still

• if the mare wants to lie down and roll, this can often be an advantage if it is proving difficult to manipulate the foal into a dorsal position

• a bridle and/or twitch may be useful but should not be relied on

• tranquillizers may make early manipulation easier, but will reduce straining when this could be helpful

• epidural anaesthesia has the same advantage and disadvantage as tranquillizers — additionally the response is slow and variable

• introduction of a stomach tube into the trachea prevents the mare from straining
• clenbuterol may help to stop mare straining
• general anaesthesia may be considered for final manipulative attempts before a surgical approach.

Manipulation
• whilst awaiting experienced help it is best to walk a mare with dystocia, to stop her from straining; this prevents further loss of fluid and reduces trauma
• vaginal examination should be made with a washed and lubricated ungloved hand — this aids the differentiation of the vaginal wall (if the cervix is closed), allantochorion and amnion
• if the allantochorion is still intact it must be ruptured using a finger (nail), guarded knife or hypodermic needle — this membrane is very tough
• if the amnion has not ruptured it is best to assess the situation, and carry out preliminary manipulations through the membrane; this prevents loss of amniotic fluid and facilitates repositioning of appendages
• initially attempts are made to ascertain the cause of the dystocia and thereafter to correct abnormalities of posture and position — the latter involves the following techniques:
 (i) repelling any part of the fetus which is in the vagina, to allow access to flexed appendages.
 (ii) application of ropes to the head and fetlocks.
 (iii) application of blunt eye hooks.
 (iv) the introduction of warm water or saline into the uterus where all the natural fluids have been lost.
 (v) applying traction to the foal, or attached ropes, once satisfactory posture and position have been achieved.
• problems encountered during manipulation are:
 (i) observers often expect rapid results and do not understand the difficulties involved.
 (ii) the mare may be uncooperative.
 (iii) pain (due to the mare straining) and tiredness of the operator's arms make manipulation progressively more difficult.
 (iv) drying of the mare's vagina makes her resentful of repeated re-insertion of the arm — it is helpful to lubricate the arm regularly but not the operative hand (which is less effective when slippery).
 (v) the ruptured amnion, particularly when trying to apply ropes

to the head, constantly insinuates itself between hand and foal, and prevents the rope from gripping.

(vi) preventing a head (which appears reluctant to be born) from flopping back into the uterus can be difficult; this probably reflects failure of the body of the foal to rotate and it may be helpful if the mare is allowed to roll.

- whilst applying traction to a foal, always consider:

 (i) is the vagina adequately lubricated?

 (ii) the direction of pull — once the fetal head is clear of the vulva the foal should be pulled towards the mare's hocks.

(iii) the strategy of traction — try to ensure that limbs are pulled alternately in unison with the mare's straining efforts — retain tension on the head.

(iv) could the fetus be oversized? — this is rare.

 (v) have the hips locked? — once the head and forelimbs are delivered the rest of the birth should be easy. If this is not so it may be because of hip lock or hind limb flexion (dog-sitting position); the latter cannot be diagnosed. In this case repel the foal if possible and rotate to a lateral position — a large rotation of the front of the foal probably only affects the hips to a minor degree — and pull again.

- when the foal is born by traction, the mare is often standing. Once the thorax starts to pass through the vulva call for assistance to support the foal to prevent trauma from falling and premature rupture of the cord (**9.5**)
- if the mare is recumbent after delivery pull the foal's forelegs round to the mare's head to establish contact
- allow the cord to rupture spontaneously; do not ligate — if haemorrhage occurs apply a haemostat temporarily
- after any delivery, particularly if it is easy, check for a twin
- the time at which manipulation and/or traction will have been considered to fail will depend on many factors, not least the possibility of quick surgical intervention.

24.5 Surgical treatment of dystocia

Embryotomy

- embryotomy involves the removal of part of the foal, *per vaginam*, either using a roughened wire or a knife
- embryotomy should only be considered in the mare if it is felt that one incision will be sufficient, or if there is no alternative

• the most likely situations when embryotomy will be applicable to the mare are:

(i) hydrocephalus — removal of the head may be facilitated by first puncturing the cranium and releasing fluid.

(ii) irreducible head/neck flexion.

(iii) where there is no alternative.

• embryotomy should never be considered if the foal is alive

• consideration should always be given to the likelihood of vaginal/uterine trauma sustained by the mare.

Caesarian operation

• this operation is elected for in cases of irreducible dystocia, or when it is considered that prompt surgery may produce a live foal

• anaesthetic and surgical procedures always pose some risk to both dam and foal, and these should not be overlooked

• the salient points of the operation are:

(i) the anaesthetic given to the mare should be one which causes minimal depression of the foal, e.g. induction with xylazine and ketamine and maintenance with halothane.

(ii) a pre-mammary gland mid-line approach is probably best.

(iii) on gaining entrance to the abdomen the uterus is immediately apparent; a recognizable part of a fetal appendage (usually a hock) should be located through the uterine wall and incised over an avascular area.

(iv) an incision of about 23 cm will allow exteriorization of first one limb (after digital rupture of the amnion) and then the other, but help will be needed to pull the foal clear of the abdomen.

(v) if possible a live foal should be held for a while, in a position which doesn't compromise the asepsis of the operation, to allow emptying of the placental vascular bed through the umbilicus; however, attempts to ensure that a potentially viable foal is breathing take precedence, and it is wise to clamp the umbilicus before severence.

(vi) contamination of the abdomen with fetal fluid, especially after a prolonged dystocia, should be minimized, although this is not always possible.

(v) after clamping any vessels in the uterine wall which are bleeding, the allantochorion is identified and peeled back from the endometrium.

NB, it may be difficult to distinguish the allantochorion from the endometrium — attempts to separate the endometrium from the myometrium will result in haemorrhage, which may be severe.

(vi) after separation of the allantochorion, the endometrium is opposed to the rest of the uterine wall, round the complete periphery of the incision, using a locking stitch.

(vii) the uterine wall is closed with a Lembert or Cushing suture, avoiding the allantochorion; if the latter membrane is included the uterus may be prolapsed during third stage labour.

(viii) after closing the abdomen, the mare should be allowed to recover sufficiently for a natural bonding to occur when the foal is presented.

(ix) as well as antibiotic and fluid therapy if required, the mare should be given a small dose (5 iu) oxytocin i.v. to aid involution and expulsion of the membranes and fluids.

(x) post-operative complications include uterine and vaginal haemorrhage, shock, wound breakdown, herniation and laminitis.

25 / The normal stallion

25.1 Anatomy (Fig. 25.1)

The scrotum

• this is the sac which contains the testes. The scrotal skin is usually hairless (except in donkeys and small ponies) and shiny

• the scrotum can change in shape to regulate the proximity of the testes to the body and thus help to control their temperature

• a septum divides the scrotum into two halves, one for each testis

• the inner lining of the scrotum (tunica vaginalis communis, or parietal layer of the tunica), is separated from the testicular covering (tunica vaginalis propria or visceral layer of the tunica) by a thin

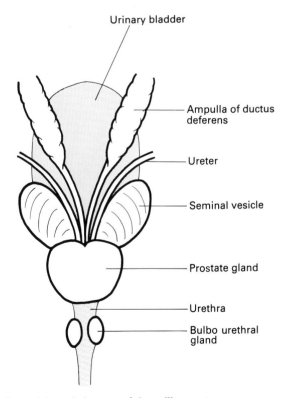

Fig. 25.1. Intrapelvic genital organs of the stallion.

film of fluid — this allows easy movement of the scrotal skin over the testis.

The testis (testicle)
- those of a thoroughbred stallion are about 10 x 6 x 5 cm; the size of the testis is roughly proportional to the size of the horse
- both testes normally are of a similar size with one lying slightly anterior to the other
- palpably the testis is firm, smooth and regular in shape
- the testis lies with its long axis horizontal

The epididymis
- a very long tube in which spermatozoa, which have left the testicle, mature
- the tube is tightly coiled upon itself and the resulting oblong structure is attached to the testis
- the head of the epididymis is on the cranio-dorsal pole of the testis
- the body of the epididymis runs caudally on the dorso-lateral aspect of the testis to the
- tail, which can be palpated on the caudal pole of the testis and is about 2½ cm³ in the thoroughbred; equine sperms are infertile until they enter the tail of the epididymis.

The spermatic cord
This is a complicated structure which contains:
- the spermatic artery
- the spermatic vein; this is spread out into a complex network of small veins (the pampiniform plexus) which surrounds the spermatic artery and cools down the blood which is going to the testis
- the cremaster muscle which can (with the scrotal skin) vary the distance of the testis from the body wall and thus influence its temperature
- the ductus deferens (vas deferens).

The ductus deferens
- this tube is a continuation of the epididymis, and transports spermatozoa from the latter to the urethra
- it enters the horse's abdomen (with the cremaster muscle, testicular vessels and their supporting tissues) through the inguinal canal

• in the abdomen the ductus deferens becomes dilated to form an ampulla, in which the sperms are stored

The inguinal canal
• this channel is formed by a gap in the abdominal muscle, just anterior to the scrotum
• soon after birth, the foal's testes should have descended through this canal and entered the scrotum; failure to do so results in a cryptorchid — if only one testis is undescended it is a unilateral cryptorchid, if both are undescended it is bilateral. The term monorchid refers to a horse with only one testicle — this is extremely rare (**28.2**)
• if the inguinal canal is too large, intestine may pass through it and cause an inguinal hernia (**27.3**); this can occur in colts or stallions or soon after castration.

The urethra
• this tube connects the opening of the urinary bladder to the tip of the penis, and conveys urine to the outside
• it also transports semen during ejaculation
• the intra-pelvic portion of the urethra is joined by three sets of glands
  (i) the prostate which partially surrounds the urethra
  (ii) a pair of large seminal vesicles which lie just on top of the bladder
(iii) a pair of smaller bulbo-urethral glands which are caudal to the seminal vesicles
• in the penis, the urethra is covered by the bulbo-spongiosus muscle, whose contractions force semen and urine along the urethra.

The penis
• this is usually housed within the sheath and is composed mainly of two erectile tissues, the corpus spongiosum penis and corpus cavernosum penis
• during erection the penis has a mechanism for filling with blood which cannot normally escape until after ejaculation
• the stallion's penis is relatively long when erect, and slightly dilated at its distal tip
• during ejaculation further swelling of the tip occurs — this dilates the mare's cervix and helps to ensure that most of the ejaculate goes into the uterus; this extra swelling can be seen if the

stallion dismounts from the mare before ejaculation is complete
• at the tip of the penis the urethra opens through the tubular
urethral process (Fig.25.2); this process is surrounded by the urethral
fossa (or fossa glandis), which dorsally adjoins a further dilation,
the urethral diverticulum. These latter two cavities are sites of
smegma accumulation.

The prepuce or sheath
This is the structure in which the inactive penis is housed.
• laterally and ventrally it is composed of skin
• internally, in the resting state, it is doubled-back on itself forming
the preputial fold; this fold straightens out during erection
• smegma also accumulates in this fold and at the base of the penis
(**26.1**).

25.2 Endocrine control

• as in the mare, the hypothalamus in the brain receives poorly
understood external stimuli, and in response produces gonadotrophin
releasing hormone (GnRH)
• GnRH acts locally on the anterior pituitary gland to allow release
of:
 (i) Luteinizing hormone (LH); in the male this hormone is also
called interstitial cell stimulating hormone (ICSH) as it travels to
the testes in the blood and there stimulates the interstitial (or
Leydig) cells to produce and release androgens and oestrogens.
(ii) Follicle stimulating hormone (FSH); the function of this hormone
is not understood, but it is thought to maintain the function of the
sertoli cells in the testis — the main role of these cells is to provide
the correct environment for developing sperms. In turn the sertoli
cells produce a hormone called inhibin which prevents excess FSH
production.
• androgens are the male hormones which stimulate the secondary
sexual characteristics of stallions and maintain their interest in
mares (libido); the stallion testis produces large amounts of testosterone, and also dihydrotestosterone and androstenedione
• *oestrogens* probably have similar functions to androgens, but it is
not known why the stallion produces such large quantities of these
hormones, i.e. 17 β-oestradiol sulphate and oestrone sulphate
• circulating blood levels of testosterone and oestrogens vary

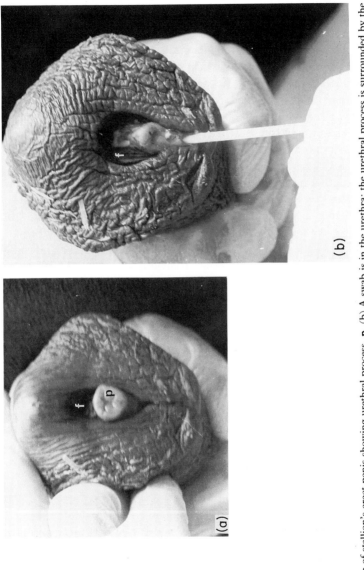

Fig. 25.2. (a) Tip of stallion's erect penis showing urethral process, **p**. (b) A swab is in the urethra; the urethral process is surrounded by the urethral fossa, **f**.

considerably from hour to hour, so that measurement of a single sample is often meaningless; concentrations (particularly oestrogens) are usually highest during the breeding season
• stallions will usually copulate all year round, but most reproductive parameters are maximal during the breeding season
• non-active stallions may have lower mean testosterone concentrations than those that are covering
• exposure of a stallion to a mare in oestrus causes a rise in circulating oestrone sulphate concentrations within ten minutes
• the reproductive season can be 'brought forward', as in the mare, by increasing artificial light; in some stallions this also produces a 'premature autumn'
• puberty, as judged by the time when the stallion's ejaculate contains a minimum of 100×10^6 sperms with at least 10% progressive motility, occurs at about 18 months; this may be influenced by the time of birth, nutritional status and breed and can be considerably delayed in certain individuals.

25.3 Physiology of sperm production

The testis is composed of a network of small tubes (the seminiferous tubules), in which sperms are formed; these tubules are supported by interstitial, or Leydig, cells which produce testosterone. The seminiferous tubules drain into the epididymis, where sperms mature; transit along the epididymis takes about 10 days.

Spermatogenesis
Spermatogenesis is the process by which sperms are formed; it basically involves multiplication of cells by division of their parents to produce the millions of sperm cells voided in each ejaculate.
• two forms of division occur:
 (i) mitosis. In this case both daughter cells are exactly the same as the parent, and it is a method by which numbers are increased.
(ii) meioisis. This is a complicated and important division in which genetic material is firstly 'shuffled', and then halved; this latter process is essential so that each sperm carries 32 chromosomes. The ovum from the mare will also contain 32 chromosomes (half the number in normal horse cells) so that combination of the two at fertilization will produce a new individual with 64 chromosomes in each cell.
• spermatogenesis is therefore a very complicated process and it is

not surprising that it sometimes goes wrong and produces abnormal cells; the whole process from parent cell to sperm, takes about 50 days.

Ejaculate
The ejaculate is the total material emitted from the stallion's penis during coitus; this is usually achieved by six to nine urethral contractions, each one producing a jet of semen (or ejaculate).
• the ejaculate is composed of:
(i) sperms (spermatozoa); there are enough sperms in the ductus deferens (including ampulla) for each ejaculation. Most of the sperms (80%) are contained in the first three jets of the ejaculate
(ii) seminal plasma; this is provided by the accessory glands (prostate, bulbo-urethral and seminal vesicles) and is the medium in which the sperms are suspended. It also acts as a temporary energy source.
• some stallions produce large quantities of a gelatinous material (gel) from the seminal vesicles; this is emitted in the latter part of the ejaculate and its function in unknown, although it can make semen evaluation difficult (**26.4**).

Normal semen
The quality of horse semen is influenced by many factors, including season of year and frequency of ejaculation. In general the higher values for the parameters measured occur in the summer in horses that are used sparingly. However, there is no clear cut link between semen quality and fertility (**27.1**)
(i) colour — pale white or skimmed milk-like; nothing like as dense as ram or bull semen.
(ii) volume 60−70 ml (30−300 ml); depends to some extent on the volume of gel.
(iii) sperm concentration — $100-800 \times 10^6$ per ml, i.e. 100 to 800 million/ml.
(iv) total sperm output (this is a more meaningful measurement than concentration) — $4-14 \times 10^9$, i.e. 4 to 14 thousand million sperms in each ejaculate.
(v) number of sperms which are able to swim in a forwards direction (i.e. progressively motile) — over 50%.
(vi) number of normal shaped (morphologically normal) sperms — over 50%.

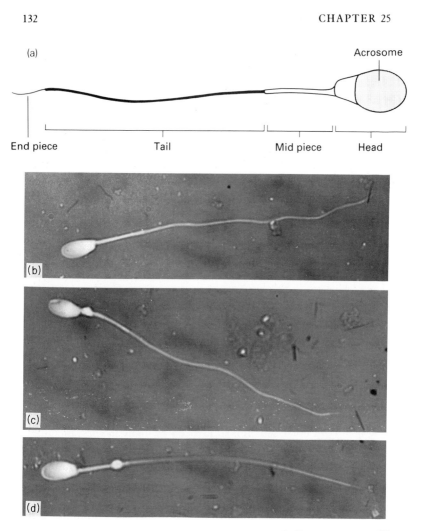

Fig. 25.3. (a) Diagram of a normal stallion spermatozoon. Stallion spermatozoa: (b) normal; (c) proximal cytoplasmic droplet and acrosomal defect; (d) distal cytoplasmic droplet and separating acrosome; (e) bent mid-piece; (f) coiled mid-piece and tail and separating acrosome; (g) knobbed acrosome.

• a normal sperm is shown in Fig. 25.3. Note that eccentric attachment of the mid piece to the head, which is abnormal in other species but acceptable in the stallion; the characteristic is described as abaxial mid-piece

• occasionally immature cells including spermatogonia are seen in the ejaculate; their effect on fertility is not known

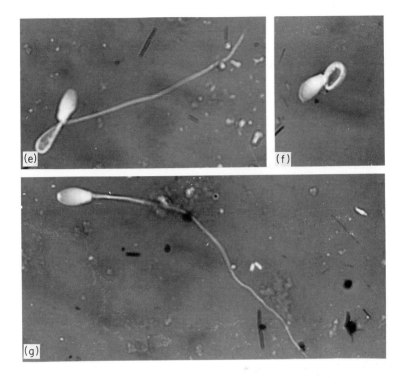

- stallions over 5 years old have greater sperm reserves than younger horses
- stallions with large testes produce more sperms
- the tail of the epididymis is the major site of sperm storage and contains more than 60% of extragonadal sperm reserves
- the rate of ejaculation does not affect sperm transit time through the epididymis.

NB, stallions with values lower than those quoted above are not necessarily infertile or sterile (**27.1**).

25.4 Covering behaviour (see also Chapter 6)

Pasture breeding
- contrary to popular belief, stallions that run constantly with mares rarely get kicked
- in the early breeding season, feral stallions tend to 'herd' their band of mares to keep them in a group

• the stallion can recognize, however, those mares that are in heat, possibly visually (by the attitude they adopt when they are near him) or by smell
• the stallion will not try to mate mares that are not in oestrus
• mares that are in heat may get covered several times a day, particularly at dawn and dusk
• stallions show a preference for some mares and may ignore other mares that are well in heat
• the restrictions on pasture breeding are that infections are hard to deal with, conception dates may be difficult to ascertain and the stallion will only be able to cover a small number of (about 15) mares.

Breeding 'in hand'

• exposure of stallions to mares only when they are ready to be covered induces a conditioned response
• usually the stallion knows when he is approaching the covering area, as opposed to being taken out to be lunged, ridden, shod etc.
• the stallion's excitement is evidenced by vocalization, rearing, bucking and trying to get close to the mare; the extent to which he becomes difficult to handle at this time depends on the individual horse, the way he has been trained and the competence of the present handler
• when confronted with a mare in heat the stallion should:
 (i) achieve an erection; this may occur before the stallion sees the mare, after a short period of vigorous 'teasing' of the mare or, in some horses, after an extremely long wait (27.4).
 (ii) tease the mare by vocalizing, licking, holding her tail in his teeth, nuzzling the vulva, nipping or biting.
(iii) exhibit flehmen, i.e. curl his lip upwards and extend his head and neck forward and upwards; stallions do this more frequently when in the presence of an oestrous, compared with a non-oestrous mare but mares, geldings and foals also do it occasionally. It is thought that this posture enhances the possibility of pherormones reaching the vomeronasal organ; sometimes mare's urine is seen to run into the stallion's nose, but often it doesn't.
(iv) mount the mare; he may try to do this immediately on contacting the mare, with or without erection, or after a variable period of teasing — correct early training is necessary to ensure that the stallion mounts at the right time.
 (v) gain intromission, followed by thrusting.

Intromission
- most stallions gain intromission without help, and some resent having their penis touched; however, help may be necessary, particularly if the mare's vulva has been stitched or is of an abnormal shape (**6.5, 13.2**) (it is essential to check that the stallion has not entered the mare's rectum)
- after gaining intromission, the stallion usually starts to ejaculate in 15–30 seconds but occasionally
- this can be almost immediate and can be missed by the handler
- some stallions dismount without having ejaculated; on average stallions require 1.5–2 mounts to achieve ejaculation.

Ejaculation
Ejaculation is recognized by:
- cessation of thrusting
- 'flagging', i.e. the stallion's tail pumps up and down; this may be difficult to recognize if the stallion is covering a tall mare as he may also be moving his tail from side to side as he shifts weight from one foot to another
- feeling urethral pulses on the ventral surface of the urethra
- observing the stallion when he has dismounted; a stallion that has ejaculated usually losses his erection and is not interested in the mare for at least a few minutes. A stallion that hasn't ejaculated usually remains keen and regains his erection rapidly (if it is lost) and re-mounts the mare. However, stallions with poor libido may lose interest without having ejaculated (**27.4**).

Dismount
- as described above, this may not indicate that the stallion has ejaculated
- if ejaculation has occurred, the stallion may dismount:
  (i) during ejaculation — in most cases the material which is lost is the viscous seminal vesicle secretion.
  (ii) after ejaculation but before loss of erection.
  (iii) after both ejaculation and loss of erection; the stallion appears to 'go to sleep'.

26 / Examination of the stallion for breeding soundness

26.1 Bacteriological swabbing (see also 14.1)

Rationale
- in most sexually transmitted bacterial diseases of horses, the stallion is purely a carrier, i.e. he shows no signs of infection and is not affected in any way
- the organisms usually thrive in the sites where smegma accumulates
- occasionally bacteria can be isolated from the internal genitalia (e.g. pathogenic Klebsiella)
- routine screening of stallions (for carriers of these venereal organisms) is therefore desirable

Requirements
- different breed societies have different requirements, and these are usually related to the value of the horses involved
- the code of practice for the control of venereal disease (Appendix 1) in the United Kingdom, Ireland and France requires that all thoroughbred stallions have two sets of swabs taken yearly, between January 1st and the start of the breeding season
- it is only logical for any stud which requires mares to have had clitoral swabs taken before covering also to have had their stallions swabbed
- a minimum requirement on any stud should be one set of swabs
- the interval of one year between swabbing is arbitary but fits in with the horse's normal breeding cycle; however, in cases of otherwise inexplicable infertility or known cases of venereal disease, extra swabs should be taken where appropriate
- the 'code of practice' recommends swabbing stallions from the urethra, urethral fossa (including the urethral diverticulum) and sheath; it also suggests collection of pre-ejaculatory fluid.

Technique
- in order to swab a stallion properly, his penis must be 'drawn' (exposed)
- this may be achieved by:

(i) administering tranquillizers, e.g. acetylpromazine, xylazine or detomidine. NB, the possibility of the stallion being unable to retract his penis after these drugs should be borne in mind and discussed with the owner before-hand. If unavoidable, xylazine is probably the drug of choice. Such a method precludes the possibility of collecting pre-ejaculatory fluid

(ii) teasing the stallion with a mare so that he achieves an erection; this may include allowing the stallion to mount an oestrous mare. The method that the author favours (finds least dangerous) is:

• have a mare, not necessarily in heat, restrained at the back of a loose box

• allow the stallion, in the yard, to tease the mare over the box door

• invariably the stallion puts his head into the doorway which reduces the likelihood of his rearing, bucking, moving sideways or observing the 'swabber'

• once the horse is drawn, even if he hasn't achieved a full erection, running the hand over the horse's side and belly and holding the penis is usually not resented

• the 'swabber', standing on the horse's left, holds the penis in his left (gloved) hand; either three swabs can be held in the right hand, each protruding through a different finger space, or successive swabs can be passed by an assistant

• passage of a swab into the urethra, and manipulation of a swab in the fossa and diverticulum are rarely noticed by the stallion

• pushing the third swab into the preputial fold, at the base of the penis, should be carried out last as this often provokes the stallion to kick

• these swabs are more likely to pick up dry material, particularly that from the prepuce, if previously moistened; this can be done by dipping into sterile water (*not* saline) or into the Amie's transport medium, before use

• swabs are immediately placed in the transport medium before being sent to the laboratory.

26.2 Physical examination

Observation

Observation of the stallion covering a mare; this is not always practical but where possible should include:

• reaction of stallion to mare — is he genuinely interested (i.e. not just noisy and physical)?
• does he gain an erection within a reasonable time?
• does he mount properly and thrust?
• can he gain intromission (given that the mare is normal)?
• does he ejaculate (as judged by palpation of the urethra)?
• does he withdraw before ejaculation is complete?

Examination of external genitalia
• penis. This is observed prior to covering — irregularities are due to haematomata or tumours
• scrotum and contents. These are more easily examined after the stallion has ejaculated; abnormalities detected may include:
(i) lesions in scrotal skin.
(ii) disparity in size of testes or epididymides (**27.3**).
(iii) abnormal position of a testis; rotation through 90 to 180° probably doesn't affect spermatogenesis and may be corrected manually.
• internal examination, *per rectum*; this is usually only carried out in cases of infertility, although routine examination, including ultrasonography, may be rewarding.

26.3 Semen collection (also see 23.1)

The artificial vagina (AV)
• several models are available, but all rely on the basic principles shown in Fig. 26.1
• most AVs have a closed collecting system, although some are open ended and semen jets have to be 'caught'
• basically there is an outer rigid tube and an inner soft liner; the space between these is filled with warm water
• the collecting system is arranged so that semen contacts the latex liner for the shortest time possible, i.e. enters the collecting vessel immediately
• in cold conditions a system of lagging the collecting vessel is desirable
• most AVs incorporate a filter (surgical gauze or double thickness tissue) which holds back the gelatinous seminal vesicle secretion, but allows passage of the sperm rich fraction (**25.3**)
NB, a significant number of sperms are lost in the liner and in the filter.

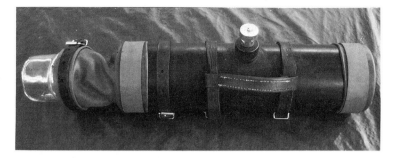

Fig. 26.1. One type of artificial vagina for collecting stallion semen.

• water at 50–52°C is introduced into the AV, to provide a temperature in the lumen of about 44°C
• the AV liner is lubricated with a non-spermicidal substance (e.g. KY jelly or vaseline — the latter is not water soluble and is difficult to remove)
• after use the liner must be cleaned meticulously, i.e. wash, rinse several times in hot running water and immerse in 70% alcohol for 20 mins; rinse with saline before use
• the temperature in the artificial vagina will fall if there is a delay in collection; ensure that more hot water is readily available should this situation arise
• assessment of the amount of water which the AV should contain is difficult if the size of the stallion's penis is not known; in general it is better to overfill the AV as water can be removed quickly and this avoids the delay of having to add more. NB, grossly overfilling the AV may cause it to disrupt
• it is essential to ensure that the hole in the collecting vessel is dorsal (to avoid spillage) and left open; otherwise air forced forward by the stallion's penis cannot escape.

Collecting a sample
• ensure that the mare holder and stallion holder know what is expected of them; consider wearing protective clothing
• select a quiet mare that is well in heat and restrain her adequately
• stand on the same side as the stallion handler (left) and allow the stallion to mount
• immediately deflect the erect penis to the side of the mare and introduce it into the AV; this may be difficult due to thrusting of the stallion and movement of the mare

• always be prepared for the mare to kick or turn, or for the stallion to dismount
• once the penis is in the AV, keep the collecting vessel lower than the other end so that ejaculate flows freely
• if the stallion is reluctant to thrust, it may be necessary for the collector to manipulate the AV over the stallion's penis
• ejaculation is recognized by appearance of fluid in the collecting vessel (if not lagged), urethral contractions or flagging
• if the stallion dismounts during late ejaculation, be prepared to let more water out of the AV to prevent the fully erect penis from sticking.
NB, temperatures in the lumen of the AV in excess of 50°C could damage sperms.

26.4 Semen evaluation

The equipment necessary for semen evaluation should have been assembled before collection, but does not need to be elaborate; basically it is essential to have a microscope, microscope slides, cover slips, pipettes, a method of keeping the sample warm (water bath), a method of keeping the microscope slides warm and vital stain, e.g. nigrosin/eosin — also of use are semen extender and buffered formal saline. The various assessments, and means by which they are evaluated are (see also 25.3):

Volume
If this cannot be measured directly from the collecting vessel the ejaculate must be transferred to a suitable (warmed) measuring device

Colour
Stallion semen is rather watery and is only likely to be discoloured by smegma and other debris, or by blood

Initial progressive motility
The vessel holding the ejaculate must be placed immediately into water at 37°C to prevent cooling — this is best achieved by using a thermostatically controlled water bath, or any vessel to which warm water can be added and its temperature checked using a thermometer.
• a drop of semen is placed (using a pipette) onto a microscope slide which is also kept warm either by housing the slide in a

thermostatically controlled stage or keeping the slide on a flat-sided medicine bottle which has been filled with warm water.
• cover the semen drop with a glass cover slip and examine under high power.
• assessment of motility is subjective, but the same observer can become very consistent; only consider sperms that are swimming across the field in a straight line — circular movement and oscillation are ignored — motility is usually assessed as 10%, 20% etc. although is rarely 100%
• diluting semen in warmed extender or 5% glucose (1:20) may give a more accurate estimation of motility as this reduces clumping, which is common in stallion semen
• the value of longivity tests is in doubt

Morphology
This is the percentage of sperms which conform to the shape accepted as normal for stallion semen
• a simple stain to use is nigrosin/eosin; this is best used soon after it is made up, and refrigerated between uses
• this stain is adequate for gross assessment of a sample, although more detailed morphology can be studied using other stains, e.g. Giemsa and by electronmicroscopy
• basically, eosin is taken up by cells that are dead at the time of staining, and they stain pink; nigrosin acts as a background so that the sperms are silhouetted against it and their shape can be seen
NB, the heads of spermatozoa are bilaterally flattened (like a table-tennis bat); in semen samples they are invariably seen lying on their widest face — in histological preparations of testes the narrow face of the head may be sectioned.
• a suggested method of preparing a vital smear is:
  (i) pipette six drops of stain into a test tube in the water bath and leave for 1−2 minutes for the temperature to equilibrate.
  (ii) add one drop of semen; this ratio will allow a sample of average concentration to provide a field with spermatozoa close enough to observe conveniently, without them lying on top of each other
  (iii) shake gently to mix, and immediately transfer one drop with a clean pipette to one of two waiting slides; smear the drop as for a blood film with a third slide and with the material left adherent to the latter make another smear on the second slide.

(iv) by experience it will become clear which smear is easier to view under the microscope, but usually it is the second.

(v) allow the smear to dry (about one minute) and assess its quality under high power (x 40 objective lens); if cells are reasonably spaced for evaluation change to oil immersion lens and record 100 cells.

NB, it is normal for the mid-piece to be attached to the side of the neck (abaxial mid piece) and stallion sperms have asymmetrical heads of varying shapes.

(vi) the main classifications of sperms will be (Fig. 25.3);

> normal — live
> normal — dead
> separated head (dead)
> knobbed acrosome
> oedematous acrosome
> detached acrosome
> crater defect
> neck tags or mid piece disruption ⎫
> proximal cytoplasmic droplet   ⎬ live
>   ⎭
> distal cytoplasmic droplet
> bent mid piece
> coiled tail
> looped tail

(vii) normal live sperm and those with a distal cytoplasmic droplet (which is a remnant of the cytoplasm left after the sperm's metamorphosis from a spermatid, and is used as an indication of sperm maturity) are added and represent the percentage of sperms which are considered normal. More detailed examination of 'normal' sperms using different stains or electron microscopy may reveal previously unrecognized abnormalities

Concentration

This can be measured using:

• an electronic counter which has been calibrated to count cells of this size

• a haemocytometer chamber

(i) well mixed semen is diluted 1:200, usually using a red cell haemocytometer pipette.

(ii) one drop is placed on the grid of the chamber, and the coverslip is applied in the recommended manner.

(iii) after focusing, the large squares (one of which just fills the field of view of a $\times 40$ objective lens) are located and the number of sperms in five of these is counted.

(iv) it is customary to count squares diagonally across the grid, i.e. squares which only contact each other by their corners; count sperms which touch the left hand and bottom lines, but not those that touch the top or right hand line.

(v) repeat the count of five squares on a different diagonal and calculate the mean for five squares; multiply the number by 10 000 to find the number of sperms/mm.^{3}

ALWAYS put some of the sample into buffered formal saline (roughly 1:1), wax the bottle cap to prevent evapouration and label the bottle clearly; this provides for retrospective checking in any cases of doubt.

NB, it has become customary to evaluate two samples collected one hour apart

27 / Infertility in the stallion

27.1 Poor semen quality

Defining the problem
- the words 'fertile', 'infertile' and 'subfertile' are all relative and describe different degrees of being able to get mares in foal
- the term 'sterile' denotes complete inability to breed, as in a castrate
- the quality of semen below which a stallion has reduced fertility cannot be defined and will, amongst other things, depend on the number of times that he is used
- it is surprising that stallions with very poor motility and/or morphology of sperms will still get a small percentage of mares in foal
- the results of semen evaluation can only be interpreted in conjunction with other information; the only proof of fertility is that the stallion covered a mare (which was not covered by another stallion at the same heat), and that she was either unequivocally found to be in foal by a method that reliably aged the pregnancy, or produced a foal at the expected time after the covering
- however, as a guideline, it has been suggested that stallions with seminal values consistently above the following should not have fertility problems; gel-free volume of ejaculate 25 ml; sperm concentration 20×10^6/ml; total sperm output 1.3×10^9; total live sperm output 1.1×10^9.

Causes
- the causes of poor seminal quality, in the absence of other obvious disease processes, are poorly understood; some possible contributing factors are:

(i) pyrexia. Any disease which causes a rise in temperature is likely to cause a disruption in spermatogenesis; however, due to antibiotics, it is unusual for such a condition to exist for any length of time. Normal sperm should appear in the ejaculate 2 months after recovery.

(ii) anabolic steroids. These drugs are most likely to be given to horses in training; they depress spermatogenesis but after withdrawal of the drug this process usually returns to normal after about 3 months.

(iii) over use. Most stallions can cover 15 times a week without a reduction of seminal quality; however, some stallions may not be able to cope with this regime — in normal stallions the third ejaculation of the day is as fertile as the first.

(iv) very rarely a stallion may produce an ejaculate of poor quality, followed 1−2 hours later by a 'normal' ejaculate; it is thus desirable to collect twice from a stallion during a fertility examination.

(v) nutritional factors may affect semen quality but these have not been described fully.

(vi) masturbation. There is no evidence that this reduces fertility.

(vii) some stallions produce a higher number of abnormal spermatozoa after a long sexual rest.

NB, it is usually suggested that semen evaluation is carried out after the stallion has rested for 5−7 days; however, for a busy stallion this may give a false impression of seminal quality

NB. The quality of the ejaculate reflects the conditions of spermatogenesis 60 days previously.

Treatment

• management. If a management factor is identified it must be corrected and if the problem appears to be recent it is worth testing again in two months

• teasing. This may decrease the reaction time and increase the volume of accessory secretion but has no effect on sperm output

• hormones. There is no evidence that hormone treatment, e.g. gonadotrophins or gonadotrophin releasing hormone, has any affect on semen quality. The use of steroid hormones is contraindicated (**27.4**).

27.2 Infections (see also Chapters 13 to 16)

General considerations

• active infection of the stallion's genital tract, giving rise to recognizable lesions, are rare (e.g. orchitis, epididymitis, seminal vesiculitis)

• two viral conditions occur, i.e. coital exanthema, which is self-limiting, and equine viral arteritis, which does not occur in the UK (see Chapter 16)

• stallions can be carriers of venereal organisms; they show no signs of disease, but spread the organisms from mare to mare. It is only this latter situation which will be considered further.

Diagnosis
• this usually occurs when pre-breeding season swabs are taken from the stallion's penis or sheath; swabs may also be taken at other times if an infectious fertility problem is suspected (**26.1**)
• the organisms which are considered dangerous are *Taylorella equigenitalis*, *Klebsiella pneumoniae* (capsule types 1, 2 and 5) and *Pseudomonas aeruginosa*
• only some strains of *P. aeruginosa* appear to be pathogenic but these cannot be identified chemically or serologically; it may be necessary to test-mate two or three mares and observe them closely for signs of endometritis
• some stallions have been known to excrete *K. pneumoniae* or *P. aeruginosa* in the ejaculate and not harbour the organism on the penis; the site of bacterial multiplication has not been found
• mycoplasmata and fungi are found in the ejaculates of many stallions but their significance is unknown

Treatment
• do not wash the stallion's penis routinely with antiseptics as these increase the incidence of resistant pseudomonads
• for stallions which ejaculate bacteria, parenteral gentamycin (4.4 mg/Kg twice daily) or neomycin (3 g/twice daily) are effective
• in general, however, systemic treatment is not necessary and the following local regime should be adopted
  (i) the stallion's penis must be exposed by teasing him with a mare, or administering sedatives (**26.1**).
  (ii) the penis and sheath must be washed thoroughly with warm water and soft soap; attention must be paid to removing smegma from the sheath and the urethral fossa and sinus.
(iii) do not use chlorhexidine; there is evidence that this can be absorbed locally and can interfere with spermatogenesis
 (iv) dry the penis well.
  (v) apply any of the following:
       an antibiotic ointment; those containing neomycin, polymyxin and furazolidine are most effective

silver sulphadiazine cream; this has been used to clear
pseudomonas organisms in particular
silver nitrate as a 1% spray
(vi) repeat the washing, drying and antiseptic routine daily for five
days
(vii) if swabs are negative for venereal organisms, a bacteriological broth containing the normal flora of the stallion's penis
(e.g. non-haemolytic streptococci, *Streptococcus faecalis*, diphtheroids etc.) is applied daily for 5 days
• if swabs are positive, cleansing treatment should be continued
• if bacteria cannot be eliminated from a stallion's ejaculate mares
can be inseminated or the minimal contamination technique used
(**15.2**)

27.3 Physical abnormalities

NB, it may be difficult to decide in some cases whether a physical or psychological problem is responsible for preventing normal
copulatory behaviour; inability to achieve normal coitus is called
impotence
• failure of both testicles to descend (bilateral cryptorchidism);
stallions with one abdominal testis (unilateral cryptorcids) are
fertile but should not be bred from (**28.2**)
• hypoplasia of both testes — rare
• atrophy or fibrosis of both testes after injury or infection — rare
• torsion of the spermatic cord — the tail of the epididymis may be
palpated in the lateral or anterior part of the scrotum; twists through
up to 180° may neither cause signs of discomfort nor infertility, and
may be reduced manually
• severe testicular torsion, and inguinal and scrotal hernias cause
acute signs of colic
• adhesions between the parietal and visceral layers of tunica vaginalis restrict movement of the testis in the scrotum and are signs
of previous damage (**25.1**)
• testicular tumours are rare, the commonest being the seminoma;
metastasis is rare
• fibrosis of the epididymis is rare and indicates previous infection
• acute orchitis, epididymitis and seminal vesiculitis are rare
• scrotal swelling is usually due to oedema, haemorrhage or hernia

• lacerations and haematomata of the penis; the horse cannot be used until these lesions have healed

• haemospermia; the source of the blood is usually the urethral mucosa — blood is seen dripping from the penis at dismount

(i) large numbers of erythrocytes cause reduced fertility by agglutinating sperms

(ii) treat with systemic antibiosis and sexual rest

• urospermia; this may be due to defective bladder sphincter control in which case urine is seen in the ejaculate intermittently:

(i) if the stallion has an overflow incontinence, urospermia is a constant feature.

(ii) the presence of urine in the ejaculate is suspected by its colour and smell (when collected with an artificial vagina) and confirmed by testing for urea and creatinine.

(iii) the presence of urine in the ejaculate does not necessarily cause infertility, even though sperms may be non-motile.

• failure to achieve an erection could be due to the presence of a stallion ring (fitted to prevent masturbation); but see also psychological infertility

• failure to ejaculate; this may also be psychological, but in some cases the stallion is thought to have ejaculated purely because he has dismounted — ejaculation can be confirmed by observing flagging, feeling urethral pulses (3 to 9), and observing the stallion after dismounting — in most cases a stallion which has ejaculated will retract his penis and show little interest in the mare, but some will mount and ejaculate again

• retrograde ejaculation — if signs of ejaculation occur but the ejaculate is incomplete, it is possible that some has passed forwards and into the bladder

• blind stallions may have problems mounting

• mounting and/or thrusting may be prevented by painful conditions, e.g. trauma, cauda equina neuritis, ilio-femoral thrombosis, laminitis, coital exanthema; the administration of analgesics may alleviate the condition

• stallion may fall off the mare before ejaculation

• overuse — this is an unlikely cause of infertility in normal stallion as:

(i) there is evidence that the first, second and third ejaculations of the day are equally fertile.

(ii) although collecting semen hourly for five ejaculations causes a decrease in volume and total sperm output, the percentage normal and motile sperms remains the same.

27.4 Psychological problems

• these account for a large proportion of infertility in stallions and usually arise because of the way the stallion has been treated
• there is often a thin line between the discipline required to manage a strong young healthy stallion, and that which acts as aversion therapy
• some stallions may have been kicked by mares, particularly when young

Signs of psychological infertility

• complete disinterest in mares, or very long reaction time; this may occur with all mares, or only some individuals, mares of a particular colour or those with foals at foot
• inability to gain an erection (suspect a stallion ring)
• inability to mount (may be physical)
• inability to thrust (may be physical). NB, if the mare has air in her vagina, e.g. after a speculum examination, a normal stallion will not be stimulated to thrust.
• inability to ejaculate after repeated thrusting and mounting
• dismounting at the beginning of ejaculation (may be physical, e.g. due to urethritis)
• inability to cover more than one mare every day or every two days
• a stallion frustrated in one of the above ways may often become very vicious towards the mare and may try to kick at the mare or handler
• some impotent stallions have normal testosterone, but lowered oestradiol, luteinizing hormone and follicle stimulating hormone concentrations — it is not known if this is cause or effect
• anabolic steroids do not reduce sexual drive.

Treatment of psychological infertility

• the therapist must be prepared to spend a lot of time with these stallions, and to be patient
• a specific diagnosis may never be arrived at, but the following suggestions may help to correct the problem:

(i) observe the stallion's behaviour with its usual handler, and then with a complete (experienced) stranger.

(ii) run the stallion with an old mare that is well in oestrus.

(iii) allow the stallion to watch another horse cover a mare that he has failed with.

(iv) restrain another horse (i.e. potential competitor) close to the problem stallion and mare; if successful this 'observer' may become a specific requirement.

(v) cover the mare's rump (particularly if the stallion shows a mare preference) with the stallion's faeces or the urine of another mare that is in oestrus.

(vi) limit the number of coverings of stallions which cannot ejaculate regularly.

(vii) diazepam, 0.05 mg/Kg intravenously, 5–10 minutes before covering has been found to be beneficial in some stallions.

(viii) placing the non-erect penis in a warm artificial vagina, even if the stallion has not mounted, may stimulate sexual arousal — this can be progressively converted into normal coital behaviour.

(ix) although in the normal stallion gonadotrophin releasing hormone administration causes an increase in luteinizing hormone, follicle stimulating hormone, testosterone and oestradiol concentrations, there is no evidence that such treatment is beneficial for impotent horses.

(x) similarly although administration of testosterone and oestradiol to geldings will restore libido, impotent stallions do not benefit from this treatment and it will adversely affect spermatogenesis.

(xi) ejaculation failure may respond to noradrenaline, e. g. 0.01 mg/kg 10–15 minutes before covering.

28 / Miscellaneous

28.1 Breeding terms

• mare owner and stallion owner can come to any agreement they like concerning the price charged for covering the mare, and the conditions which apply to payment of the fees

• it is always wise for both stallion owner and mare owner to be clear about the terms, and to sign documents which outline the agreement

• where applicable, the stage at which a mare is certified in foal, e.g. 40 days, should be stated; irrespective of historical consideration the aforementioned is a convenient time to define pregnancy for physiological reasons (**17.5**)

• as part of the agreement, the stallion owner may promise to restrict the number of mares covered by the stallion during the relevant season

• the stallion owner may also reserve the right to refuse nominations to certain mares, e.g. maiden and old barren mares

• some examples of agreements are set out below:

(i) straight fee. This becomes payable at the end of the breeding season (15th July for thoroughbreds) provided that the mare has been covered.

(ii) split fee. Part of the payment is due at the end of the breeding season (whether or not the mare is certified in foal); the remainder becomes payable either on 1st October if the mare owner cannot produce a certificate from a veterinary surgeon to say that the mare is not in foal, or at a specified date if the mare does not produce a foal which lives for 7 days.

(iii) in some cases split fees which are due on 1st October offer an extra incentive for those who pay promptly in respect of the mare producing a viable foal (length of survival post-partum is defined).

(iv) no foal — no fee: a mare not in foal on October 1st evokes no stud fee. In some cases the stud returns the fee if no live foal is born.

(v) no foal, free return provides that should a mare fail to produce a foal which lives to a specified age, the mare will be covered again by the same stallion in the next year, but thereafter renewal of the 'free return' is unlikely.

28.2 The 'riggy' gelding

The problem
• the word 'rig' is one which is applied to cryptorchid horses, which have one or both testes undescended (still in the abdomen) (**25.1**)
• occasionally horses that are considered to be geldings may have one (in this case the other, descended, testis has been removed by castration) or both testes in the abdomen; although these testes cannot produce sperms, they do produce male hormones and the horse acts like a stallion
• many geldings are said to be 'riggy' because they exhibit behaviour which is interpreted as stallion like, or because they are difficult for the owner to manage
• the sort of behaviour that evokes the description of 'riggy' includes:
 (i) chasing or 'herding' mares or other horses in a field.
 (ii) obtaining an erection either in the presence of other horses or otherwise.
(iii) aggression towards other horses, particularly stallions and colts.
(iv) mounting mares in heat, with or without an erection.
 (v) covering mares.
(vi) biting objects, people or other horses.

Possible causes of 'riggy' behaviour
• retention of one or both abdominal testes — this can be diagnosed by hormonal tests — see next section
• cutting the horse proud, i.e. castrating the horse by removing the testis but leaving either the epididymis or a lot of the cord; this does *not* produce a true rig because:
 (i) many horses castrated in this way do not exhibit the above behaviour.
 (ii) growing cells from the epididymis and cord in the laboratory (tissue culture) shows that they are incapable of producing male hormones (testosterone and oestrogens).
(iii) horses which have deliberately been castrated to leave the epididymis intact do not give positive responses to the hormone tests for true cryptorchids.
(iv) however, removal of the cord from previously castrated horses will sometimes improve behaviour; the mechanism by which this works is not known

• Age of castration

(i) in a study on the behaviour of castrated stallions, most showed a marked lack of interest in mares by 30 days after the operation.

(ii) in a different study which compared the behaviour of geldings that were either castrated before 2 years of age, or after 3 years of age, it was found that in both groups 30% of the horses were less aggressive to people and 40% were less aggressive to other horses, i.e. the age of castration had no effect on aggression. NB, this means that most geldings show some signs of aggression — and so do many mares; often the problem is managemental, including lack of confidence by the owner.

Fertility in 'rigs'

• horses with no testes cannot be fertile

• cryptorchid horses are also sterile; although the testes in the abdomen can produce hormones, the temperature is too high for spermatogenesis

• after castration horses are usually sterile by 7 days; sperms may remain in the ampullae for several months but these are invariably dead.

Diagnosis of the 'true rig' (cryptorchid)

Two hormonal methods are available: these are easier and cheaper than surgical exploration of the abdomen.

• testosterone: concentrations of this hormone vary so much that a single sample will not give an interpretable result

(i) it is therefore necessary to inject the horse with a hormone which will, if normal testicular tissue is present, stimulate exaggerated testosterone production.

(ii) the test procedure is: take a heparinized blood sample for resting plasma testosterone concentration determination: inject 6000 i.u. human chorionic gonadotrophin (hCG) intravenously: take a second blood sample for testosterone determination 30 to 120 minutes after injection — a significant elevation in testosterone in the second sample indicates the presence of testicular tissue (interstitial or Leydig cells).

• oestrone sulphate — a single blood sample taken into a herparinized container will allow assay of plasma oestrone sulphate concentrations; high values indicate the presence of testicular tissue. NB, this latter test is not suitable for horses under 3 years of age or for donkeys.

28.3 Stallion 'vices'

• so called vices in stallions, as in other horses, are usually caused by the boredom that results from being confined to a loose box for most of the day
• these include box walking, weaving, crib-biting, wind-sucking, kicking, etc.
• where stud management allows, stallions should be ridden, lunged or even turned out into a small paddock daily
• well exercised stallions are much easier to handle when covering
• the use of stallion rings to stop masturbation or prevent erections during showing etc. is to be avoided if possible.
NB, some stallions are evil; so are some mares and some geldings.

28.4 Hidden costs at stud

• when sending your mare to stud, the covering fee is not the only expense that will be incurred
• incidental costs may be negligible compared with the stud fee, but the following should be anticipated:

Keep fees
These are increased if the mare has a foal at foot and should be balanced carefully with the possible benefits of travelling the mare to and from the stud and of obtaining veterinary advice.

Transportation costs
These must be incurred for travelling the mare to and from the stud once. However, if the mare is collected and taken home after covering and returned for pregnancy tests etc., these trips should be costed.

Management costs (i.e. routine worming and foot care)
All studs must adopt a sensible worming programme and your mare cannot be an exception; it is contamination of pasture which is the greatest danger to your mare (and particularly her foal).

Routine veterinary costs
Each stud adopts its own policy of vaccination against equine influenza, equine herpes virus, and tetanus — additionally prebreeding

genital swabbing is usually required, and newborn foals may receive antibiotics, tetanus antitoxin and regular examinations.
• these measures are part of the intense preventive medicine regime that studs must adopt in order to try to safeguard all of the animals on the premises — your mare and/or foal cannot be an exception
• attention post-foaling, i.e. examination of membranes, suturing the vulva etc.

Specialist veterinary costs
These include:
• examination for breeding soundness
• additional uterine swabs
• examination for failure to show heat
• examination to assess readiness for covering
• prescription of hormone injections or other preparations
• treatment of uterine infections
• pregnancy diagnosis, either manual or with ultrasound (these may need to be repeated)
• management of twins.

Emergency veterinary costs
These are likely to be incurred during parturition problems or any other disease which affects either the mare or the foal.

28.5 Rectal tears

• examination of the mare's genitalia *per rectum*, either by palpation or ultrasound scanning, is the most commonly employed gynae-cological investigation
• this method of examination is also frequently used in horses of all types for the investigation of other abdominal conditions, e.g. colic and cryptorchidism
• a small, but real danger in all these examinations is that the horse's rectum may become torn often with fatal consequences.

Some facts concerning rectal tears
• compared with the number of horses which are examined *per rectum*, damage to the rectum wall is very infrequent
• rectal tears occur more often in male horses than females; this may be because:

(i) mares become accustomed to rectal examination; but every animal must be examined for a first time.

(ii) stallions and geldings may be more difficult to restrain during examination.

(iii) male horses may have more 'fragile' rectums than females.

(iv) the reason for rectal examination in male horses, e.g. crypt-orchidism may require more extensive abominal exploration.

(v) in emergencies, e.g. colic, it is more likely that mares will have been previously examined by this method than male horses

• rectal tears happen most often during examinations by experienced practitioners

• rectal tears rarely occur in the area where the examiner's fingers are placed, i.e. adjacent to the structure being palpated; commonly they occur on the dorsal surface of the rectum, adjacent to the mesorectum, i.e. the lesion results from pulling the rectum away from its mesenteric attachment

• examiners are often unaware of rectal tears occurring, probably because they occur at the back of the hand

• because the usual site for rectal tears is about 30 cm cranial to the anus, and at the site of dorsal rectal attachment, it has been postulated that a weakness exists in this area in some horses

• rectal tears can occur spontaneously.

Possible causes of rectal tears

• application of excessive pressure to the rectal wall — this cannot be quantified but it is unlikely that an examiner will consciously evoke a rectal tear

• resentment of examination by the horse — during every exam-ination the hand experiences various degrees of rectal pressure caused by involuntary peristalsis or voluntary straining; during mild peristaltic contractions examination can be continued; during strong peristaltic waves the hand should be left immobile and passive until the contraction has passed; during forceful abdominal straining the hand should be retracted and occasionally withdrawn from the rectum. NB, rarely, conditions may be such that a com-plete examination cannot be carried out in an uncooperative animal; re-examination later, or on the next day is usually less complicated, although economical and practical considerations may make re-examination difficult.

• sudden movements of the animal which cannot be anticipated —

restraint during rectal examination is discussed in Chapter 3 and the degree adopted is usually sufficient for the examiner to feel safe. However, sudden events which may scare the mare cannot be prevented, e.g. an attendant sneezing, a car starting, a dog barking, a foal moving etc.
• predisposing weakness of the rectal wall because of previous lesions or unknown factors

Recognition of rectal tears
• many rectal tears occur unknown to the examiner
• signs which may make the examiner suspicious that a rectal tear has occurred are:
(i) a sudden increase in space in the rectum — this could be due to air entering the rectum from the colon or through the anus
(ii) the presence of blood on the examiner's sleeve; usually this is the result of a minor abrasion of the rectal wall or damage to the anus — in the vast majority of cases it is inconsequential. If blood is seen, a *careful* re-examination should be made; unless the examiner is aware of the usual site for rectal tears (this is unlikely to happen to any clinician more than once in his/her lifetime) a dorsal tear may be missed.

Treatment of rectal tears
Once a diagnosis has been made, treatment is aimed at preventing fatal peritonitis and includes:
• antibiosis
• analgesia when required
• fluid therapy if necessary
• attempts at surgical repair of the rectum are heroic and have not been shown to improve the prognosis.
NB, the consequences of rectal tears are rarely modified significantly by treatment and severe ruptures usually result in death of the horse due to peritonitis or adhesions.

Appendix / A Common Code of Practice for the Control of Contagious Equine Metritis and other Equine Reproductive Diseases for the 1987 Covering Season in France, Ireland and the United Kingdom*

*Published by the Horserace Betting Levy Board, November 1986. Reprinted by permission of the editor of the *Veterinary Record*.

Recommendations to mare and stallion owners for the 1987 covering season

Introduction
1 The recommendations continue to be the minimum requirements for the examination of mares and stallions and it is emphasized that owners should consult their veterinary advisers concerning the implementation of the Code. As more information becomes available amendments to the Code may be introduced.

Definitions
2 The definitions used in this appendix are as follows:

(A) *High risk mare*

(i) All mares from which the CEMO has been isolated on a previous occasion.

(ii) A mare covered by a stallion which transmitted CEM in 1986

(iii) All mares arriving from countries other than France, Ireland and the United Kingdom or covered by stallions resident in countries other than France, Ireland and the United Kingdom during 1986.

Information with regard to the identity of high risk mares may be obtained from the appropriate authority.*

(B) *Low risk mare*

All mares not included in (A) above.

(C) *Swabs*

(i) Mares

(*a*) Endometrial swab — A swab taken during early oestrus from the lining of the uterus.

(*b*) Clitorial swab — A swab taken from the clitoral fossa including the clitoral sinuses using a swab suitable to penetrate the clitoral sinuses.

(ii) Stallions

(*a*) A sample of the pre-ejaculatory fluid.

(*b*) A swab taken from the penile sheath.

(*c*) A swab taken from the urethra.

(*d*) A swab taken from the urethral fossa.

All swabs should be immediately despatched to a Designated Laboratory and be cultured under both microaerophilic and aerobic conditions so that the presence of the CEMO and other pathogens may be identified and subsequently reported. Microaerophilic cultures for CEM should be incubated for a minimum of six days although the laboratory may issue a preliminary report at four days if requested.

France: Syndicat des Eleveurs de Chevaux de Sang de France, 76 Champs Elysees, 75008 Paris (tel. 225 25 15).

Ireland: The Irish Thoroughbred Breeders' Association, Johnstown, Naas, Co. Kildare (tel. 045 97459).

UK: The Thoroughbred Breeders' Association, Stanstead House, The Avenue, Newmarket, Suffolk (tel. 0638 661321).

Recommendations to mare owners

All mares

3 Owners should compile a detailed history of their mares whilst at stud in 1984, 1985 and 1986 and the information should be entered on the Mare Certificate. This should include the results of positive bacteriological tests undertaken including tests for the CEMO since 1977. If the mare is examined prior to being moved to the stallion stud farm, the results should be entered on a laboratory certificate. The stallion stud farm should receive the Mare Certificate and, if applicable, the laboratory certificate before the mare is moved.

Requirements

4 (A) *High risk mares*

(i) Prior to going to the stallion stud farm, one negative clitoral swab.

(ii) On arrival at the stallion stud farm, one negative clitoral swab.

(iii) On the stallion stud farm, one negative set of endometrial and clitoral swabs should be taken during the oestrus prior to covering.

(iv) Mares to be walked in may be swabbed at the boarding stud by arrangement with the Stallion Stud management.

(B) *Low risk mares*

(i) One negative clitoral swab. This may be taken either at the stallion stud farm or on the home stud farm providing there is agreement with the stallion stud manager.

(C) *All mares*

(i) On the stallion stud farm prior to covering an endometrial swab should be taken during oestrus and cultured aerobically to identify other bacteria capable of causing venereal disease.

Abortion

5 If abortion occurs the foetus and placenta should be sent to a laboratory which regularly carries out equine post-mortem examinations and the mare put immediately into isolation until it is shown to be free from any identified infection.

In-foal high risk mares

6 In-foal high risk mares should be foaled in isolation with hygienic disposal of the placenta. In addition to the recommendations in 4A, a cervical swab should be taken at foaling or within 12 hours of foaling. Foals born to these mares should be swabbed on three occasions at intervals of not less than seven days before they reach three months of age. Filly foals should be swabbed in the clitoral fossa and colt foals should be swabbed inside the penile sheath and around the tip of the penis.

Recommendations to stallion owners

All stallions and teasers

7 Stallions and teasers should be subjected to examination and swabbing of the external genital organs by a veterinary surgeon. The examination should be carried out after 1st January 1987 but before the start of the covering season. A set of swabs should be taken on two occasions at not less than seven days interval and the results of their examination entered by the veterinary surgeon on the Stallion Certificate. As an additional precaution the first mares covered by a first season stallion should be thoroughly screened for evidence of CEM as determined by the stud farm veterinary surgeon; the number to be screened will be at his discretion. The stallion owner or stud manager will then be able to inform owners of mares booked to a particular stallion of the results of the tests.

Hygiene

8 It is important that all personnel realize the highly contagious nature of CEM. This especially applies to pregnant mares known to be infected with CEM. Personnel should always wear disposable gloves when handling the external genitalia of mares and stallions.

Walking in mares

9 (A) *Low risk mares*
On the first occasion before each mare is walked-in , a clitoral swab should have been taken before the mare goes to the stallion stud farm. An aerobic endometrial swab should also be taken during oestrus. Additional swabbing should be done at the discretion of the stallion stud manager and the attending veterinary surgeon. In doing so they should liaise with the veterinary surgeon responsible for the mare.
(B) *High risk mares*
When high risk mares are walked in they should be boarded at a farm;
 (i) Under the control of the stallion stud farm, or
(ii) Which meets the full approval of the stallion stud farm management and their veterinary advisers.

In the case of (ii) there should be close liaison between the relevant veterinary practices to ensure that the recommendations of the Code and any additional precautionary measures in operation on the stallion stud farm itself are satisfied.

If CEM is confirmed on the boarding stud farm where the mare resides or on the stallion stud farm which it has visited, no mare should be moved from the boarding stud farm until all mares at the boarding stud farm have been swabbed with negative results.

The examination of mares after covering has commenced

10 If in the opinion of the attending veterinary surgeon an abnormal pattern of returns to service develops it is imperative that a full set of swabs is obtained and cultured under aerobic and microaerophilic conditions.

Action if CEM or other venereal disease occurs

11 The action to be taken when CEM is confirmed is as follows
   (a) Mares prior to covering
      (i) Isolate and treat infected mares as advised by the attending veterinary surgeons
      (ii) Notify all owners of mares booked to the stallion(s) including those which might have already left the stallion stud farm.
      (iii) Notify the appropriate authority.*
   (b) Mares and stallions after covering: Apply (i), (ii), and (iii) as above and in addition:
      (iv) Cease covering by the stallion which should be swabbed and treated as advised. Covering should not resume until the stallion has been treated and has had three negative sets of swabs taken at intervals of not less than two days. The first swab should not be taken until at least seven days have elapsed after treatment is completed.
      (v) Check and deal with all mares which are implicated in the outbreak as advised by the veterinary surgeon and blood samples should be taken 19–40 days after service and sent to a laboratory which can carry out the tests. (Information about these tests can be obtained from the appropriate authority as in paragraph 11, (a) (iii).)
12 The action to be taken when other venereal diseases are confirmed:
   (i) mares — isolate and treat infected mares as advised by the attending veterinary surgeons.
   (ii) stallions — cease covering. The stallion should be swabbed and treated as advised. Advice on the resumption of covering will be given by the attending veterinary surgeon.

---

*France: Service des Haras, 14 Avenue de la Grand Armee, Paris.
Ireland: Equine Section, Veterinary Research Laboratory, Abbotstown, Castleknock, Co. Dublin (tel. 01 213041).
UK: The Thoroughbred Breeders' Association, Stanstead House, The Avenue, Newmarket, Suffolk (tel. 0638 661321).

Export certification

13 All swabs taken for export of horses should be sent to Ministry of
Agriculture, Fisheries and Food Laboratories for culture.

Certification

14 Certificates may be obtained from the following on receipt of a large
stamped addressed envelope:

France: Syndicat des Eleveurs de Chevaux de Sang de France, 76 Champs
   Elysees, 75008 Paris.

Ireland: The Irish Thoroughbred Breeders' Association, Johnstown, Naas,
   Co. Kildare.

United Kingdom: The Thoroughbred Breeders' Association, Stanstead
   House, The Avenue, Newmarket, Suffolk.

Rhinopneumonitis virus abortion

1 Characteristics of the disease

Rhinopneumonitis abortion is caused by a virus of the herpes group, equid
herpes virus 1, Sub-type 1 ($EHV1_1$). The equid herpes 1 variant, Sub-type
2 ($EHV1_2$), causes respiratory disease only. Rhinopneumonitis abortion
virus ($EHV1_1$), is readily destroyed outside the body by heat and disinfectants,
but if cleaning and disinfection are not adequate the virus may survive for
several weeks.

The virus can cause a mild fever, coughing, nasal discharge and other
signs of respiratory infection, usually in weaned foals and yearlings. The
respiratory form of the disease occurs most frequently in autumn and
winter. However, infection of the respiratory tract and excretion of virus
may occur without clinical signs of illness.

This virus causes abortion in mares in late pregnancy, usually between
8 and 11 months of gestation, *but it can be as early as 5 months*. Abortion
can occur from two weeks to several months after infection. Field obser-
vations suggest that prolonged transport and other types of stress during
late pregnancy may increase the likelihood of infection of the fetus.

At full term, a foal may be born alive but infected. Such foals are
usually abnormal from birth, with signs of weakness, jaundice or difficulty
in breathing. They are highly infective, and virus is likely to be shed freely
into the environment. Usually death occurs in one to three days but
occasionally foals survive longer.

2 Means of spread

Aborted fetuses, fetal membranes and fluids are a dangerous source of
infection but mares may also acquire infection from horses and foals

excreting the virulent strains of virus as aerosol from the respiratory tract. Carrier mares and other horses exhibiting no clinical symptoms may be a source of infection.

After virus abortion or the birth of an infected foal, the virus does not appear to persist long in the mare's genital tract. The respiratory tract of aborted mares is, however, a potential source of infection to in-contact mares.

3 Diagnosis

The disease can be diagnosed by post-mortem examination of the fetus or foal and the detection of characteristic microscopic changes in the tissues. Confirmation of the diagnosis may be provided by virological examination of the tissues. This usually requires one to two weeks. Serological examinations alone are not a suitable means of diagnosis.

4 Prevention and control of equine rhinopneumonitis

It must be remembered that any recommendations for the control of virus abortion are inevitably a compromise between procedures that are scientifically desirable and those that are practicable for the industry.

A Management

(i) Where practicable, mares should be foaled at home and sent to a stallion with a healthy foal at foot

(ii) When this is not possible, the mares should be sent to the stallion stud at least one month before foaling is due and put into group isolation. Ideally these groups should be as small as possible. Mares in late pregnancy which have come from sales yards or from abroad constitute a particular risk and should be separately isolated.

(iii) Pregnant mares should be segregated as far as possible from weaned foals, yearlings, horses out of training, hunters and competition horses. If handled by the same attendant, the work schedule should be arranged to allow the mares to be handled first.

(iv) There is a risk in transporting mares in late pregnancy with other stock. In particular they should not be travelled with recently aborted mares.

(v) If a *foster mother* has to be brought on to a stud where pregnant mares reside, she should be strictly isolated until the possibility of her own foal's death being due to rhinopneumonitis is excluded.

B Isolation facilities

Isolation facilities should be provided at all studs to prevent the spread of rhinopneumonitis and other infections. The design and construction should be undertaken in consultation with the stud's veterinary surgeon, who should also be consulted about the precautions to be taken to prevent the spread of infection by the attendant.

C Disinfection
It is essential that routine and regular cleansing of horse conveyances is carried out in accordance with regulations of the respective Ministries of Agriculture, Fisheries and Food.

D Vaccination
An inactivated rhinopneumonitis vaccine is presently available for the control of the disease and mare owners should consult their veterinary surgeon about its use and regarding a suitable vaccination programme. Vaccination programmes formulated to provide protection against rhinopneumonitis virus abortion should not by themselves be allowed to engender a false sense of security. It must be stressed that vaccination cannot replace sound management practices which should be arranged in consultation with the studfarm veterinary surgeon.

Action to be taken when abortion, stillbirth or birth of a sick foal occurs
(i) Action should be taken in the case of any abortion, stillbirth or foal death within seven days of birth, even if the mare concerned is believed to have been vaccinated against rhinopneumonitis. The stud's veterinary surgeon must be notified immediately and arrangements made, on his advice, for appropriate investigations to be undertaken. The fetus or foal and its membranes should be sent to a recognized centre for post-mortem examination. The possibility of virus infection should also be considered when the foal is ill at birth. If the foal is alive but possibly infected, a diagnosis may be made by virological examination of nasopharyngeal swabs taken from the foal. These should be submitted to an appropriate laboratory as soon as possible.

(ii) The mare should be in strict isolation pending results of the examinations. All bedding should be sprayed in the box with disinfectant and left for 48 hours; it can be removed and burned at a later date. The box should then be washed and liberally soaked with a disinfectant such as one of the Iodophor group and the box thoroughly cleansed with water under pressure or steam according to the instructions of the stud's veterinary surgeon.

(iii) No horse should be removed from the stud premises until the possibility of rhinopneumonitis abortion has been excluded.

(iv) If preliminary laboratory investigations are indicative of rhinopneumonitis infection, close contact pregnant mares should be divided into small groups as soon as possible to minimize the spread of infection. Despite these precautions some of these mares may still abort.

(v) If rhinopneumonitis abortion is subsequently confirmed at a stud, the appropriate Breeders' Association* should be notified immediately. At the same time owners or their agents with mares at the stud, or due to send mares there, should be informed. Those studs to which mares from the infected premises have been, or are to be, sent should also be informed.

(vi) Notification of cases to the Breeders' Association is of the utmost importance to the long-term interests of all owners of mares. No stigma is attached to an abortion attributable to rhinopneumonitis on a stud, but failure to notify the disease leads directly to the spread of infection to the detriment of all owners and their horses, especially mare owners.

(vii) Any foal which is ill at birth or becomes unwell within seven days of birth should be carefully examined by a veterinary surgeon.

6 Subsequent action

(i) Providing there is no sign of infection at home, barren and maiden mares, and mares which have foaled at home and produced normal healthy foals, can be accepted on the stud on which a confirmed virus abortion has occured.

(ii) These mares (enumerated in (i) above) can leave the stud at which the abortion has occurred after one month from the date of the last mare to abort at the stud, provided they are subsequently isolated from in-foal mares for at least two months.

(iii) The infected stud's own non-pregnant mares can visit other premises after one month from the date of the last abortion, provided they can be isolated for at least two months from heavily pregnant (more than five months) mares at the stud they are visiting. Full agreement on these arrangements should be reached between the home stud and the receiving stud and their respective veterinarians. Pregnant mares must remain on the infected stud until they foal.

(iv) Present evidence indicates that there is little risk of spread of infection if a mare is covered on her second heat cycle after abortion. It is emphasized that she must be isolated from mares in late pregnancy for eight weeks after abortion.

(v) Mares that have returned from studs where rhinopneumonitis virus abortion has occurred during the previous season should be foaled *in isolation* at home.

France: Syndicat des Eleveurs de Chevaux de Sang de France, 76 Champs Elysées, 75008 Paris (tel. 225 25 15).
Ireland: The Irish Thoroughbred Breeders' Association, Johnstown, Naas, Co. Kildare (tel. 045 97459).
UK: The Thoroughbred Breeders' Association, Stanstead House, The Avenue, Newmarket, Suffolk (tel. 0638 661321).

Further reading

Ginther, O.J. (1979) *Reproductive Biology of the Mare*. Equiservices, 4343 Garfoot Road, Cross Plains, Wisconsin 53528.

Ginther, O.J. (1986) *Ultrasonic Imaging and Reproductive Events in the Mare*. Equiservices, 4343 Garfoot Road, Cross Plains, Wisconsin 53528.

Males, R. & Males, V. (1977) *Foaling: Brood Mare and Foal Management*. Landsdowne Press, Sydney.

Pickett, B.W., Squires, E.L. & Voss, J.L. (1981) *Normal and Abnormal Sexual Behaviour of the Equine Male*. Animal Reproduction Laboratory, Colorado State University, Fort Collins, Colorado 80523.

Rossdale, P.D. & Ricketts, S.W. (1980). *Equine Stud Farm Medicine*, 2nd Edition. Bailliere Tindall, London.

Walker, D.F. & Vaughan, J.T. (1980) *Bovine and Equine Urogenital Surgery*. Lea & Febiger, Philadelphia.

Zemjanis, R. (1970) *Diagnostic and Therapeutic Techniques in Animal Reproduction*, 2nd Edition. The Williams and Wilkins Company, Baltimore.

Index

Abortion 90−1
  bacterial causes 94
  equine herpes virus 1 (EHV1) 88,
    95, 164−7
  miscellaneous causes 98
  practice code 161, 166−7
  twins 37, 97−8
  viral infections 95−7, 164−7
  see also Pregnancy, failure
Allanto-chorion 33, 104−109,
Allyltrenbolone
  anoestrous shortening 22
  ovulation synchronization 24
Anabolic steroids
  puberty effects 8
  spermatogenesis effects 144−5
Androgens 128, 130
Androstenedione 128
Anoestrous 6, 18
  transition 6, 18
    erratic 55−6
    shortening 22−3
  see also Oestrous, absence
Arteritis, viral 88
Artificial insemination (AI) 114−16
  advantages 114
  disadvantages 144−15
  semen collection 115
  semen treatment 116

Bacteraemia, pregnancy failure 94−5
Bacterial infections
  infertility 53−7
  pregnancy failure 94−5
Breeding
  additional costs 154−5
  'in hand' 134−5
  pasture 133−4
  terms of agreement 151
Bridle, mare restraint 10
Broad ligaments 2
Bulbo-spongiosus muscle 127
Bulbo-urethral glands 127

Caesarian section, dystocia 123−4
Caslick's operation 12, 65−6
Cervix 1−2
  adhesions 61, 69

cyclical changes 18−21
  fibrosis 61, 69
  pregnancy changes 36
  rupture 111
Chorio-allantoic membrane (see
  allanto-chorion)
Chorio-allantoic pouches 31, 105
Chromosome abnormalities 59−60
Clinical examination
  Clinician's approach 11−12
  examination per rectum 13
  examination per vaginum 14
  external examination 12
  mare restraint 9−11
Clitoral sinusectomy 86, 87
Clitoral swabbing 71−3, 160−2
Clitoral winking (showing) 25
Conception, rates 52
Conceptus
  definition 89
  development 30, 31−2
Contagious equine metritis (CEM)
  69−70, 146
  clitoral swabbing 71−3, 160−2
  penile swabbing 136
  practice code 159−67
  speculum examination 73−8
  uterine swabbing 73−9
Corpus cavernosum 28, 127
Corpus haemorrhagicum (CH) 4, 19,
  20
Corpus luteum (CL)
  development 20
  formation failure 16, 57
  persistent 21, 55
  ultrasonic appearance 16
  progesterone 34−5
  regression 35, 36
Corpus spongiosum 127
Covering
  injuries 28−9
  mare restraint 26−7
  stallion behaviour 133−5
Cremaster muscle 126
Cryptorchidism 147, 152−3
Cysts
  endometrial 14, 41, 60, 84−5
  fossa 58

ovarian, misdiagnosis 57—8
para-ovarian 58

Dihydrotestosterone 128
Dioestrous *see* Interoestrous
Dismount, post-coital 135
  semen sample 115
Ductus (vas) deferens 126—7
Dysmaturity 38, 93
Dystocia 49, 118—24
  Caesarian section 123—4
  definition 118
  embryotomy 122—3
  manipulation, *per vaginam* 121—2
  recognition 119—20
  restraint 120—1
  significance 119
Ejaculate
  composition 131
  stallion 131
  see also Semen; Sperm
Ejaculation 135
  failure 148
  noradrenaline effects 150
  retrograde 148
Embryo
  definition 89
  development 14, 34, 42
  micromanipulation 117
  resorption 90
  transfer 117—18
Embryotomy 122—3
Endometritis
  causes 82—85
  chronic, treatment 84
  cystic, treatment 84—5
  prostaglandin production 68
  swabbing techniques 71—81
  treatment/prevention 82—7
Endometrium, biopsy 79—81
Epididymis 126
Equine chorionic gonadotrophin
    (PMSG) 34
  normal pregnancy 31, 34, 36
  pregancy diagnosis 41, 43
Equine herpes virus 1 (EHV1)
  abortion 88, 95, 164—7
  diagnosis 95—6, 165
  epidemiology 96
  infection control 96, 164—6
Equine herpes virus 3 (EHV3) 88
Exanthema, coital 88
Export certification 164

Fallopian (uterine) tubes 5

Fertility 52—4, 144
  management effects 52—4
  'riggy' geldings 153
  see also Infertility; Subfertility
Fetal membranes
  development 32—4
  examination 104—5
  expulsion 47, 48
  retention 105—9
Fetus
  definition 89
  development 13, 35
  mummification 37, 90
  position/posture 118—19
  presentation 118
  resorption 90
Flehmen 134
Foal, sick, practice code 166—7
Foal heat 50—1
  failure 56
Foal scour 50, 51
Foaling rates 52
Follicle stimulating hormone (FSH) 8
  male 128
Fossa cysts 58

Geldings, 'riggy' 152—3
Genetic engineering 117
Genital tract, mare, cyclical
    changes 18—21
Genitalia
  anatomy 1—5
  bacteriological swabbing 9—18
  external examination 12
  stallion, anatomy 125—30
    bacteriological swabbing 136
    clinical examination 137
    ultrasound examination 137—17,
      40—42
Gestation, variable duration 44—5
Glands (also see pregnancy)
  urethral 127
Gonadotrophin releasing hormone
    (GnRH) 128
  ovulation effects 24
Granulosa cell tumour 58, 59

Haematomas
  penile 28
  post-ovulation 59
  post-partum 111—12
Haemospermia 148
Hobbles, mare restraint 10, 26, 27
Human chorionic gonadotrophin (hCG)
    24

Hunter Improvement Scheme   52
Hymen, persistent   61−2
Hypocalcaemia, post-partum   113
Hippomanes   33−4

Induction of parturition   47−9
    complications   49
    indications/criteria   47
Infections
    bacterial   63−70, 94, 108−9, 160−4
    post-partum   50
    viral   88, 95−6, 164−7
Infertility, mares
    infections   50, 63−7, 94, 160−4
    non-infectious causes   55−62
    viral causes   88, 95−7, 164−7
Infertility, stallion   144−50
    infections   145−7
    physical abnormalities   147−9
    psychological problems   149−50
    semen quality   144
Inguinal canal, stallion   127
Inhibin   128
Interoestrous (dioestrous)   6, 20
Intersex   59−60
Interstitial cell stimulation hormone
    (ICSH)   128
Intromission   27−28, 135

Klebsiella pneumoniae   69, 71, 146

Labour
    first stage   45−6
    second stage   46−7
    third stage   47, 48
Laminitis, placenta retention   106
Lighting, anoestrous shortening   22−3
Luteal phase
    oestrous cycle   8
    shortening   23−4
Luteinizing hormone (LH)   8
    males   128

Mare, covering injuries   28−9
Meiosis   130
Mesosalpinx   4, 5
Mesovarium   2
Metritis   85, 106
Mitosis   130
Mummification, fetal   37, 38, 90

Noradrenaline, ejaculation effects   150
Nymphomania   58

Oestrogens   8

male synthesis   128, 130
    pregnancy   36, 43
Oestrus   6, 18−20
    absence, pregnancy   39
    detection   25
    post-partum   50−1
    signs   25
    split   57
Oestrous cycle
    artificial control   22−4
    endocrine control   6−8
    genital tract changes   18−21
    hormonal changes   8
    length   6
Ovaries   2, 4
    cyclical changes   16, 18−21
    cystic, misdiagnosis   57−8
    pregnancy changes   36−7
    tumours   59
'Overdue' foal   38, 44−5
Ovulation   7, 19
    CL formation failure   16, 57
    induction   24
    synchronization   24
Oxytocin, parturition induction   47

Pampiniform plexus, spermatic artery
    126
Para-ovarian cysts   58
Parturition
    endocrine control   44
    environment preparation   44
    induction   47−9
Pasture breeding   133−4
Penis   127−8, 138
    injuries, post-coital   28
    swabbing   136
Perineum, parturition trauma   110−11
Placenta   32−3
    expulsion
        abnormal   105−9
        normal   104
    oestrogens, pregnancy   43
    retention   104−9
        membrane examination   104−5
Placentitis, pregnancy failure   94
Pneumovagina (wind sucking)   64−7,
    84
    Caslick's operation   64, 65−6
    Pouret's operation   66−7
    treatment   85
Post-partum behaviour, erratic   56
Pouret's operation, pneumovagina
    66−7

Practice codes (1987), CEM and
    reproductive disease   159−67
Pregnancy
    clinical examination   40
    conceptus development   30, 31−2
    diagnosis   39−45
    duration   37−8
    extended   38, 44−5
    failure   91−3 (see also Abortion and
        Resorption)
    uterine changes   30−1
Prematurity   93
Prepuce (sheath)   128
Progesterone   8, 20
    effect of infection   68
    pregnancy levels   34−5, 39−40
Prolonged dioestrus   21, 55, 57
Prostaglandins   6−8
    luteal phase shortening   23−4, 68
    ovulation synchronization   24
    parturition induction   47
    side-effects   24
Prostate   127
Pseudomonas aeruginosa   63, 69, 71, 87,
    146
Pseudopregnancy   58, 91, 99−100
Psychological infertility
    signs   149
    treatment   149−50
Puberty   8
    stallion   130
Pyometra   68−9
    treatment   85
Rectal tears
    causes   156−7
    examination-associated   155−7
    male/female incidence   155−6
    recognition   157
    treatment   157
Recto-vaginal fistula   65, 110
Rectum, genitalia examination
    manual   12−13, 40
    ultrasound   13−17, 40−41
Reproductive disease, practice code
    159−67
Reproductive function, investigation
    methods   54
Resorption, embryo/fetus   90
Restraint
    clinical examination   9−11
    dystocia treatment   120−1
    mare covering   26−7
Rhinopneumonitis *see* Equine herpes
    virus
'Riggy' geldings   152−3

Scrotum   124−5
Semen
    collection   138−40
        AI   115
    colour   140
    concentration   142−3
    dismount sample   115
    evaluation   140−3, 144−5
    morphology   131−3, 141−2
    motility   140−1
    quality   144−5
    treatment, AI   116
    volume   140
    see also Ejaculate; Sperm
Seminal plasma   131
Seminal vesicles   127
Seminiferous tubules   130
Septicaemia, pregnancy failure   94−5
Silent heat   39, 51, 56−7
Specula, types   15−17
Speculum examination   9, 14, 73−8
Sperm, normal   131−3, 140−3
    see also Ejaculate; Semen
Spermatic artery, pampiniform plexus
    126
Spermatic cord   126
Spermatogenesis   130−3
    anabolic steroid effects   144−5
Spermatogonia   132
Stallions
    covering injuries   28
    external genitalia, examination   138
    infertility   144−50
    physical examination   138−9
    puberty   130
    reproductive anatomy   125−30
    'vices'   154
Sterility   144
Stillbirth, practice code   166−7
Stocks, mare restraint   9−10
Straw/hay bales, mare restraint   10
Stud fees
    additional costs   154−5
    agreement   151
Subfertility   144
    chromosome abnormalities   60
Swabbing, stallion   136−7
    technique   136−7

Taylorella (Haemophilus) equigenitalis
    (see contagious equine metritis)
Teasing/teasers   26
    practice code   162
Teratomas, ovarian   59

Testes 126
   abnormalities, infertility 147,
      152−3
Testosterone 128, 150
Training, puberty effects 8
Turner's syndrome 59
   immaturity misdiagnosis 8
Twinning 17, 37
   diagnosis 101−2
   infertility 101−3
   management 102−3
   pregnancy failure 97−8
Twitch, mare restraint 10, 11, 26

Udder, post-partum engorgement 113
Ultrasound scanning
   genitalia 13−14, 15, 16, 17
   pregnancy diagnosis 40−1, 42
   twinning 102
Urethra, stallion 127
Urethral process, stallion 128, 129
Urospermia 148
Urovagina, treatment 84
Uterine (Fallopian) tubes 5
Utero-ovarian ligament 2
Uterus 2, 3
   body 2, 3
   cysts 60
   horns 2, 3

partial dilation 60
post-partum involution 50
pregnancy changes 30−1
prolapse, post-partum 112
rupture 111
swabbing 73
   bacteriological culture 78−9
   cytological examination 78
torsion 99

Vagina 1
   artificial (AV), semen collection
      115, 138−40
   injuries, post-coital 28−9
   manual examination 17
   rupture 111
   visual examination 14−17
Vaginal bleeding 62
Vas deferens 126−7
Venereal metritis 69−70, 87, 160−4
Ventral hernia 99
Vestibule, genital 1
Viral infections 88, 95−7, 164−7
Vulva 1
   parturition trauma 110
Vulvo-vaginal constriction 1

Wind sucking see Pneumovagina
Wry-neck 119